Marine Anti-inflammatory Agents 2020

Marine Anti-inflammatory Agents 2020

Editors

Donatella Degl'Innocenti
Marzia Vasarri

MDPI • Basel • Beijing • Wuhan • Barcelona • Belgrade • Manchester • Tokyo • Cluj • Tianjin

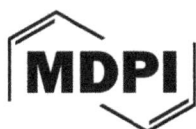

Editors
Donatella Degl'Innocenti
Università degli Studi di Firenze
Italy

Marzia Vasarri
Università degli Studi di Firenze
Italy

Editorial Office
MDPI
St. Alban-Anlage 66
4052 Basel, Switzerland

This is a reprint of articles from the Special Issue published online in the open access journal *Marine Drugs* (ISSN 1660-3397) (available at: https://www.mdpi.com/journal/marinedrugs/special_issues/Anti-inflammatory2020).

For citation purposes, cite each article independently as indicated on the article page online and as indicated below:

LastName, A.A.; LastName, B.B.; LastName, C.C. Article Title. *Journal Name* **Year**, *Volume Number*, Page Range.

ISBN 978-3-0365-0788-0 (Hbk)
ISBN 978-3-0365-0789-7 (PDF)

© 2021 by the authors. Articles in this book are Open Access and distributed under the Creative Commons Attribution (CC BY) license, which allows users to download, copy and build upon published articles, as long as the author and publisher are properly credited, which ensures maximum dissemination and a wider impact of our publications.

The book as a whole is distributed by MDPI under the terms and conditions of the Creative Commons license CC BY-NC-ND.

Contents

About the Editors vii

Preface to "Marine Anti-inflammatory Agents 2020" ix

Adrian Florian Bălașa, Cristina Chircov and Alexandru Mihai Grumezescu
Marine Biocompounds for Neuroprotection— A Review
Reprinted from: *Mar. Drugs* 2020, *18*, 290, doi:10.3390/md18060290 1

Joon Ha Park, Ji Hyeon Ahn, Tae-Kyeong Lee, Cheol Woo Park, Bora Kim, Jae-Chul Lee, Dae Won Kim, Myoung Cheol Shin, Jun Hwi Cho, Choong-Hyun Lee, Soo Young Choi and Moo-Ho Won
Laminarin Pretreatment Provides Neuroprotection against Forebrain Ischemia/Reperfusion Injury by Reducing Oxidative Stress and Neuroinflammation in Aged Gerbils
Reprinted from: *Mar. Drugs* 2020, *18*, 213, doi:10.3390/md18040213 25

Tran Minh Ha, Dong-Cheol Kim, Jae Hak Sohn, Joung Han Yim and Hyuncheol Oh
Anti-Inflammatory and Protein Tyrosine Phosphatase 1B Inhibitory Metabolites from the Antarctic Marine- Derived Fungal Strain *Penicillium glabrum* SF-7123
Reprinted from: *Mar. Drugs* 2020, *18*, 247, doi:10.3390/md18050247 39

Qingchi Wang, Weixiang Liu, Yang Yue, Chaomin Sun and Quanbin Zhang
Proteoglycan from *Bacillus* sp. BS11 Inhibits the Inflammatory Response by Suppressing the MAPK and NF-κB Pathways in Lipopolysaccharide-Induced RAW264.7 Macrophages
Reprinted from: *Mar. Drugs* 2020, *18*, 585, doi:10.3390/md18120585 55

Thilina U. Jayawardena, K. K. Asanka Sanjeewa, Hyo-Geun Lee, D. P. Nagahawatta, Hye-Won Yang, Min-Cheol Kang and You-Jin Jeon
Particulate Matter-Induced Inflammation/Oxidative Stress in Macrophages: Fucosterol from *Padina boryana* as a Potent Protector, Activated via NF-κB/MAPK Pathways and Nrf2/HO-1 Involvement
Reprinted from: *Mar. Drugs* 2020, *18*, 628, doi:10.3390/md18120628 71

Laura Micheli, Marzia Vasarri, Emanuela Barletta, Elena Lucarini, Carla Ghelardini, Donatella Degl'Innocenti and Lorenzo Di Cesare Mannelli
Efficacy of *Posidonia oceanica* Extract against Inflammatory Pain: In Vivo Studies in Mice
Reprinted from: *Mar. Drugs* 2021, *19*, 48, doi:10.3390/md19020048 87

About the Editors

Donatella Degl'Innocenti obtained a Ph.D. in Biochemistry, and she has been Associate Professor of Biochemistry in the Department of Experimental and Clinical Biomedical Sciences "Mario Serio" (University of Florence, Italy) since 2001. During her scientific career, she built national and international scientific collaborations. She is an active researcher and the leader of her department laboratory (https://www.sbsc.unifi.it/vp-223-gruppo-degl-innocenti.html). She has strong, independent research experience with an impact in the field, as demonstrated by several publications as senior author in international peer-reviewed journals. She is also a member of the Scientific Committee of the Interuniversity Center of Marine Biology and Applied Ecology (CIBM) of Livorno (Italy). In recent years, she has focused her research on the health role of natural and marine compounds. She studied the amyloid aggregation process and potential inhibitory mechanisms of natural compounds and the extract of a Mediterranean red seaweed. Prof. Degl'Innocenti has also studied the biological properties of extracts obtained from the leaves of the *Posidonia oceanica* (L.) Delile marine plant, focusing on the role of these extracts on pathophysiological cellular processes, such as inflammation and oxidative stress, but also on cancer cell migration and protein glycation processes.

Marzia Vasarri has been a Ph.D. student in Biomedical Science at the Department of Experimental and Clinical Biomedical Sciences "Mario Serio" (University of Florence, Italy) since 2017. She obtained a Bachelor's degree in Biotechnology in 2014 and a Master degree in Medical and Pharmaceutical Biotechnology in 2016. During her studies, she acquired technical-scientific skills in biochemistry and molecular biology. Her Ph.D. research investigates the bioactive properties of phytocomplex from the marine plant *Posidonia oceanica* in different in vitro cellular models. Her research focuses on exploring the role of *P. oceanica* phytocomplex on a variety of pathophysiological cellular processes, from inflammation and oxidative stress to tumor cell migration and protein glycation processes, and its potential as an inducer of the autophagy process. Her research interest also includes the field of neurodegeneration and amyloid aggregation process, as demonstrated by published works on the anti-amyloidogenic activity of the red Mediterranean seaweed *Halophytis incurva* and the protective role of Maysin against amyloid cytotoxicity. She has also conducted research on the biological properties of natural products delivered within nanosystems capable of improving the efficacy and bioavailability of the encapsulated compound in order to exploit its full potential.

Preface to "Marine Anti-inflammatory Agents 2020"

Inflammation is a finely regulated defensive response against pathogens, toxic agents, cellular injury, or tissue damage, aimed at evading or removing harmful stimuli and restoring tissue homeostasis. However, when the response is not controlled, inflammation can lead to the pathogenesis of various diseases. The need to find new and potent anti-inflammatory compounds has encouraged the scientific community to explore the marine environment as a promising source of bioactive compounds. The unique chemical diversity of marine-derived molecules represents a strategic goal for natural drug discovery against inflammation-related diseases.

This Special Issue covers original and innovative basic research regarding the anti-inflammatory potential of several classes of secondary metabolites (i.e., polyphenols, phytosterols, proteoglycans, and polysaccharides) in manifestations of acute and chronic inflammation in both in vitro and in vivo experimental models.

For the first time, the anti-inflammatory and analgesic role of a hydroalcoholic extract from leaves of the *Posidonia oceanica* marine plant was shown in a model of acute inflammatory pain in vivo; this activity was attributable to the synergistic action of its constituents, mainly represented by polyphenols.

Furthermore, beneficial effects of fucosterol from *Padina boryana* were highlighted in a model of particulate matter-induced inflammation in macrophages; while the LPS-induced inflammation model in macrophages was used to demonstrate the anti-inflammatory role of a proteoglycan isolated from Bacillus sp. BS11 (EPS11) or metabolites from the Antarctic marine-derived fungal strain *Penicillium glabrum* (SF-7123).

Another work shows that laminarin, a polysaccharide isolated from brown algae, is able to protect neurons from ischemic brain injury in in vivo models of adult gerbils by attenuating IR-induced oxidative stress and neuroinflammation.

This Special Issue includes a review that accurately describes the neuroprotective effects of important marine-derived bio-compounds.

Ongoing global research on the bioactivities of marine agents undoubtedly represents a sustainable innovation in the field of natural health products.

Donatella Degl'Innocenti, Marzia Vasarri
Editors

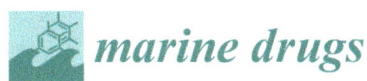

Review

Marine Biocompounds for Neuroprotection—A Review

Adrian Florian Bălașa [1], Cristina Chircov [2] and Alexandru Mihai Grumezescu [2,3,*]

[1] Târgu Mureș Emergency Clinical Hospital, "George Emil Palade" University of Medicine, Pharmacy, Science and Technology of Târgu Mureș, RO-540142 Târgu Mureș, Romania; adrian.balasa@yahoo.fr
[2] Faculty of Applied Chemistry and Materials Science, University Politehnica of Bucharest, RO-060042 Bucharest, Romania; cristina.chircov@yahoo.com
[3] Research Institute of the University of Bucharest (ICUB), University of Bucharest, 060101 Bucharest, Romania
* Correspondence: grumezescu@yahoo.com; Tel.: +40-21-402-39-97

Received: 11 May 2020; Accepted: 28 May 2020; Published: 31 May 2020

Abstract: While terrestrial organisms are the primary source of natural products, recent years have witnessed a considerable shift towards marine-sourced biocompounds. They have achieved a great scientific interest due to the plethora of compounds with structural and chemical properties generally not found in terrestrial products, exhibiting significant bioactivity ten times higher than terrestrial-sourced molecules. In addition to the antioxidant, anti-thrombotic, anti-coagulant, anti-inflammatory, anti-proliferative, anti-hypertensive, anti-diabetic, and cardio-protection properties, marine-sourced biocompounds have been investigated for their neuroprotective potential. Thus, this review aims to describe the recent findings regarding the neuroprotective effects of the significant marine-sourced biocompounds.

Keywords: marine biocompounds; neuroprotection; neurodegeneration; Alzheimer's disease; Parkinson's disease

1. Introduction

Considering their co-evolution with the associated biological targets, natural products have been favored by scientists for drug discovery and development in the treatment of various human diseases [1,2]. In this context, natural compounds represent the main treatment strategy for 87% of human diseases [3], with 63% of the newly developed drugs being categorized as naturally derived, either modified natural products, unmodified natural products, or synthetic products with a natural compound as the pharmacophore. Moreover, approximately 68% of all anti-infectious drugs, including antibacterial, antiviral, antifungal, and antiparasitic compounds, and 63% of anti-cancer drugs used between 1981 and 2008 were obtained from natural sources [4]. The advancements in the field of natural products are based on their considerable impacts on the pharmaceutical interests and the associated economic activities. Thus, there is a high interest in the discovery of small drug molecules from templates and designs of biologically and chemically diversified natural product pools, the development of novel separation, purification, and characterization techniques and the establishment of test scaffolds [5–7]. In this manner, sampling understudied locations of the planet to enhance the knowledge in the biogeography area is fundamental [8].

While terrestrial organisms represent the primary current source for developing natural therapeutics, there has been an increasing interest in focusing on marine organisms [1]. As oceans occupy more than 70% of the earth's surface, their biodiversity is a source of various types of micro- and macro-organisms offered by different oceanic zones, which makes them an essential reservoir of natural products [4,9–11]. The marine environment, through the use of fish and algae, has represented a source of medicines and oils since ancient times [4,12,13]. The increased marine biodiversity is a result of the different conditions in terms of pressure, temperature, salinity, illumination and nutrient levels, and oxygen and ion concentrations that lead to specific adaptations and specializations of the organisms [1,9,14,15]. Organisms can be found at all depths, from planktonic organisms in the upper ocean and fish and marine mammals that inhabit deeper waters, to benthic organisms that can be found throughout the ocean basins, even at the bottom of the Mariana Trench, 10,900 m below the sea level [16]. Considerable efforts in studying natural marine compounds began in 1951 through the isolation of spongothymidine and spongouridine from the sponge *Cryptotethya crypta* Laubenfels, which led to the synthesis of the anti-cancer agent arabinosyl cytosine [10]. With the advances in deep-sea sample collection, scuba diving, and novel techniques for drug development and aquaculture, an essential number of marine-derived compounds have been discovered and applied for various therapies [11,17]. Subsequently, marine organism exploitation started with collecting large creatures, including red algae, sponges, and soft corals. It continued with microorganism exploitation, such as marine bacteria and cyanobacteria and marine fungi that can produce structurally diverse metabolites [10,15].

The continuously growing interest in marine-derived biocompounds can be justified by the structural and chemical properties that are not usually found in terrestrial products, with several bioactive marine-sourced natural molecules exhibiting considerable bioactivity ten times higher than terrestrial-sourced molecules [1,4,14]. Therefore, marine plants, animals, and lower organisms represent a valuable source of biocompounds, with 650 compounds isolated in 2003, and 3000 active molecules out of 13,000 described currently [4,9,18]. In this manner, marine pharmacology is continuously proving its potential in the biomedical field through the biological functions of the most intensively studied biocompounds, i.e., carbohydrates, polyphenols, peptides, proteins, pigments, and essential fatty acids, which include antioxidant, anti-thrombotic, anti-coagulant, anti-inflammatory, anti-proliferative, anti-hypertensive, anti-diabetic, and cardio-protection properties [18]. In this manner, this review aims to highlight the main bioactive compounds currently used in the biomedical field, with a particular emphasis on the neuroprotective effects of these biocompounds.

2. Neurodegenerative Disorders and Mechanisms of Neuroprotection

Neurons continuously require high levels of energy for maintaining protein and organelle quality control, rapid molecule delivery in and out of cells, and transferring organelles and other factors throughout the cell. Since they cannot divide, an impairment of the pathways involved in these functions will subsequently lead to neurodegeneration [19]. Neurodegeneration is a complex progressive multifactorial process that leads to the loss and death of neuronal structures in the nervous system [20]. Mainly occurring in the later stages of life, neurodegeneration is associated with the accumulation of insoluble deposits of protein and peptide aggregates and inclusion bodies in different areas of the brain and spinal cord. These deposits generally contain misfolded proteins, molecular chaperones, and ubiquitin, E3 ligases, and proteasome subunits as components of the ubiquitin–proteasome system [19,21]. Neurodegeneration implies additional underlying mechanisms, such as oxidative stress, calcium deregulation, mitochondrial dysfunction, axonal transport deficits, abnormal neuron–glial interactions, neuroinflammation, DNA damage, and aberrant RNA processing [20]. Consequently, such processes gradually overwhelm the self-defense mechanisms, leading to life–death imbalances and culminating in programmed cell death through several death paths, including apoptosis, necrosis, autophagy, and parthanatos [22].

Hence, neurodegenerative disorders are accompanied by structural, chemical, and electrophysiological abnormalities in the brain and spinal cord, causing muscle weakness, poor coordination, seizures, pain, permanent paralysis and loss of sensation, and cognitive performance alterations and dementia. There is a wide range of neurodegenerative diseases that pose major concerns among aging populations worldwide, including Alzheimer's disease (AD) and Parkinson's disease (PD) as the most prevalent ones [20,23–26]. While certain genes give rise to disease-specific protein inclusions, there is common pathobiology that supports the efficiency of similar therapy strategies for various neurodegenerative diseases [19].

AD is the most common neurodegenerative disorder and the predominant form of dementia among the elderly. With approximately 44 million people living with AD or related dementia and nearly 5 million new cases reported annually, the numbers are expected to double by 2030 and triple by 2050 [27–29]. AD is characterized by an abnormal accumulation of amyloid-β proteins as amyloid plaques and hyperphosphorylated tau proteins that form intracellular neurofibrillary tangles. These processes consequently lead to synapse dysfunction and loss, inflammatory responses, and neuronal loss and microtubule disassembly, dendritic collapse, and axonal degeneration, respectively [21,27,29,30]. PD is the second most common neurodegenerative disease, with 273 per 100,000 individuals between the ages of 50 and 59, and 2700 per 100,000 individuals between 70 and 79 [28,31]. PD is a chronic disorder characterized by the progressive degeneration of dopaminergic neurons in the substantia nigra pars compacta and the accumulation of cytoplasmic inclusions and α-synuclein-containing Lewy bodies [21,31,32]. Clinically, PD is a multisystem disorder with both neurologic and systemic manifestations, including unilateral rest tremor, bradykinesia, rigidity, and disordered balance, gait, and falls [31,33]. As current treatments only help to relieve some of the physical and mental symptoms, there is no available cure. With continuous health improvements, there is an increased life expectancy worldwide. Consequently, as there is a greater risk for developing an age-related neurodegenerative disease, novel, and efficient strategies to ensure neuroprotection are fundamental [28].

Neuroprotection is a mechanism that aims to counter the process of neurodegeneration and brain malfunctioning through chemical, genetic, biological, physiological, or behavioral interventions, which could affect pathophysiological or compensatory adaptive neural mechanisms [34]. Subsequently, since spontaneous neural regeneration in the central nervous system does not generally occur, and the neuroplasticity mechanism is usually insufficient, additional strategies must be implied [35]. In this regard, a series of biomaterials in the form of nanoparticles or scaffolds have been investigated for their neuroprotective and neuroregenerative capacities [23], including alginate, gelatin, collagen, chitosan, hyaluronic acid, and poly(lactic-co-glycolic acid). Their use as microcarriers for the release of neuroprotective molecules has the potential to satisfy the therapeutic necessity for pharmacological release by reducing the degradation susceptibility and activity decay and, therefore, extending their action [36,37]. Recent years have witnessed a great focus on the discovery of natural substances with neuroprotective potential that could be efficient in the prevention and/or treatment of neurodegenerative disorders [38]. As oxidative stress has been considered to play an essential role in the onset and progression of neurodegeneration, there has been a significant scientific focus on the development of antioxidant compounds for neuroprotection [39]. The importance of the marine environment as a source of pharmaceutical agents targeting the central nervous system has been demonstrated through various studies regarding the neuroprotective and neuroregenerative effects of marine biocompounds. Thus, the following sections focus on describing the characteristics of such biocompounds and the most recent studies regarding their neuroprotection potential. For this review, the biocompounds were selected based on recent studies from 2018–2020, which have identified potential neuroprotective activities either as neuroprotective bioactive compounds themselves or as carriers for the delivery of drugs for neuroprotection.

3. Marine Polysaccharides for Neuroprotection

Marine organisms are highly rich in carbohydrates, especially in the form of sulfated and non-sulfated polysaccharides (Table 1, Figure 1) [40]. Chitin is described as a family of polysaccharides composed of linear β-(1,4)-2-acetamido-2-deoxy-D-glucose or N-acetylglucosamine [41–44]. Chitin, the second most abundant natural polymer of the ecosystem after cellulose [42,44–46], represents the main component of the exoskeleton of marine arthropods and crustaceans, especially shrimps, crabs, lobsters, krill, oysters, prawns, and squid [41–45,47]. While it is mainly extracted from the fishing industry waste, some fungi, mollusks, and nematodes can also be a source [43–45]. Chitin is obtained as a colorless or off-white powder that is insoluble in aqueous media or polar solvents due to its high cohesive energy caused by strong intermolecular hydrogen bonds formed between amide bonds [41,44,45]. Chitin is mainly used for producing chitosan, which is the partial or full alkaline deacetylation product of chitin [41,43,48–50]. In this manner, during the deacetylation process in the presence of sodium hydroxide, the acetyl bonds are broken to form glucosamine [43], and a linear polysaccharide with randomly distributed β-(1,4)-linked D-glucosamine and N-acetyl-D-glucosamine is formed [42,45,49,51–53]. Many studies have reported biocompatibility, biodegradability, non-toxicity, immunomodulatory, anti-tumor, antioxidant, hypolipidemic, neuronal regulatory, and anti-microbial properties of chitosan, which highly depend on the degree of deacetylation and the polymer chain size, i.e., an 87 kDa chitosan proved to be more effective than a 532 kDa chitosan against bacterial strains and a lower deacetylation degree leads to a higher degradation rate and host inflammatory response [42,43,48,51,52,54,55]. A wide array of studies investigated the potential of chitosan for neuroprotection. In this manner, chitosan nanoparticles have proved their therapeutic effects on BV-2 glial cells, an immortalized rat microglial line that mimics the characteristics of primary microglia, exposed to hydrogen peroxide [56]. Similar results were obtained using chitooligosaccharides on SH-S5Y5 neurons after exposure to hydrogen peroxide, with the highest activity at the lowest concentration of 0.02 mg/mL [57]. Furthermore, carboxymethylated chitosan protected Schwann cells against hydrogen peroxide-induced damage and apoptosis, resulting in decreased lactate dehydrogenase release and enhanced cell viability through the mitochondrial-dependent pathway [58]. Additionally, similar studies were performed using protocatechuic acid-grafted chitosan and rosmarinic acid-loaded chitosan nanoemulsions on neuron-like rat phaeochromocytoma cells and rat astrocyte primary cultures, respectively. Both studies showed promising neuroprotective effects against hydrogen peroxide and L-glutamic acid-induced apoptosis and LPS-induced oxidative stress [59,60]. Moreover, the neuroprotective effects of chitosan were investigated on PD models. Specifically, low molecular weight sulfated chitosan proved its potential to reduce the consequences of the disease on rotenone-treated SH-SY5Y cells [61]. Similarly, rotigotine- and naringenin-loaded chitosan nanoparticles showed alleviated effects of 6-hydroxydopamine-induced neurotoxicity in SH-SY5Y cells [62,63]. Additionally, rotigotine administration to haloperidol-induced PD rats led to decreased lactate dehydrogenase and increased catalase activities, as well as catalepsy reversal, akinesia, and swimming ability restoration [63]. Beneficial effects have also been shown against multiple sclerosis, using dimethyl fumarate-loaded chitosan nanoparticles on rodent models that led to significantly increased locomotion scores [64]. Another study proved the repair potential of LINGO-1–directed siRNA-loaded chitosan nanoparticles on demyelinated rat models with compromised motor performance and coordination [65]. Additionally, chitosan scaffolds have been shown to give a high nerve fiber regeneration capacity when compared to alginate or chitosan–alginate scaffolds in spinal cord injury rat models [66].

Table 1. The sources of the main marine-derived polysaccharides.

Biocompound	Marine Sources
Chitosan	shrimps, crabs, lobsters, krill, oysters, prawns, and squid
Alginate	brown algae (*Laminaria hyperborea*, *Laminaria digitata*, *Macrocystis pyrifera*, *Ascophyllum nodosum*, and *Laminaria japonica*)
Carrageenan	red edible algae of the *Rhodophyceae* class (*Chondrus crispus*, *Kappaphycus alverezii*, *Eucheuma denticulatum*, and *Gigartina stellate*)
Fucoidan	brown algae (mozuku, kombu, limu moui, bladderwrack, and wakame)
Laminarin	brown seaweeds (*Laminariaceae*, *Laminaria*, *Saccharina*, and *Eisenia* species)

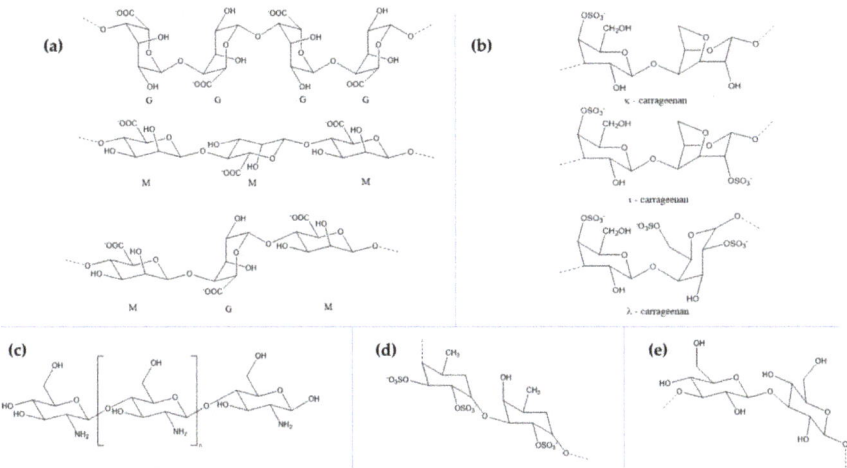

Figure 1. The sources of the main marine-derived polysaccharides: (**a**) alginate; (**b**) carrageenan; (**c**) chitosan; (**d**) fucoidan; (**e**) laminarin

Marine flora has received increasing interest as a source for marine polysaccharides due to their abundance, unique physicochemical properties, and low extraction costs [67]. Marine algae represent an ideal candidate for extracting polysaccharides owing to their various biological properties, including antioxidant, antiviral, antibacterial, anticancer, anti-inflammatory, immunomodulation, blood coagulation, hypolipidemic and hypocholesterolemic, and osteoprotective effects, which are crucial for pharmaceutical and biomedical research [40,67–70]. They cannot be found elsewhere [71]. The essential seaweed-derived polysaccharides with neuroprotective effects are alginate, carrageenan, fucoidan, and laminarin [67–69,71].

Alginate, the term generally used for alginic acid salts and derivatives, but also for alginic acid itself, is a natural linear polysaccharide consisting of β-(1,4)-linked D-mannuronic acid and α-(1,4)-linked L-guluronic acid units [72–76]. Consequently, the polymeric backbone consists of homogenous sequences of mannuronic acid (M) or guluronic acid (G) blocks, and alternating sequences (MG) [72,77,78]. Since β-1,4 linkages confer a 4C1 chair conformation that imparts flexibility to the chain and α-1,4 linkages lead to a 1C4 conformation, which is considerably stiff, the stiffness of the backbone blocks decreases in the order GG, MM, and MG [72]. Alginate is extracted from brown algae, where it exhibits structural functions as a cell wall component, comprising about 30% dry weight. Most common sources of alginate are *Laminaria hyperborea*, *Laminaria digitata*, *Macrocystis pyrifera*, *Ascophyllum nodosum*, and *Laminaria japonica* [72–75,77,79,80]. Alginate is usually extracted through the dissolution of seaweed biomass with a basic solution, precipitation in calcium chloride, filtration, purification, and drying steps [75,80]. The physicochemical properties of alginate, such as gel formation or viscosity, are directly influenced by the ratio of mannuronic to guluronic acid, the arrangement and length of the blocks, and the molecular size of the polymers, which differ depending on the isolation source or the extraction season [72,75,77]. One research group investigated the neuroprotective effects of seleno-polymannuronate prepared from alginate-derived polymannuronate. Their results suggested that this biocompound exhibited increased mitochondrial membrane potential and inhibition of amyloid-β aggregation and reduced APP and BACE1 protein and cytochrome c expression in N2a-sw cells, proving its potential in preventing neurodegeneration [81]. Moreover, ellagic acid-loaded calcium–alginate nanoparticles were administered to male Swiss albino mice with pentylenetetrazol-induced seizures. Results showed the superior effects of this system, which prevented increased glutamate, decreased γ-aminobutyric acid concentrations, and ameliorated increased amyloid-β and homocysteine levels [82]. Similarly, erythropoietin–alginate microspheres administered in Balb/c-strain mice improved locomotor and glutathione peroxidase activity, with no significant differences when using increased polymer concentrations [83]. Furthermore, paclitaxel-encapsulated poly(lactic-co-glycolic acid) microspheres embedded in alginate hydrogels provided a sustained drug delivery system in spinal cord injury models [84].

Carrageenan comprises a family of hydrophilic high molecular weight biopolymers consisting of linear sulfated galactans [85–90]. These galactans are composed of D-galactose and 3,6-anhydrogalactose residues linked through alternating α(1,3) and β(1,4) glycosidic bonds [88,91–93]. Carrageenan contains a repeated and alternating structure of 1,3-linked β-d-galactopyranose and 1,4-linked α-d-galactopyranose units [87,94,95]. Depending on their structural features, such as sulfate patterns or 3,6-anhydrogalactose presence on D-galactose units, there are at least 15 distinct types of carrageenans [91,95]. However, owing to their gelling and viscoelastic properties, κ-, ι-, and λ-carrageenan are of commercial importance [89,92–96]. Carrageenan is isolated from the extracellular matrix of red edible algae of the Rhodophyceae class [88–90,94,95,97]. While the original source was *Chondrus crispus*, the extensive use of carrageenan has led to the introduction of novel species. Specifically, κ-carrageenan and ι-carrageenan are produced from warm-water seaweeds, namely *Kappaphycus alverezii* and *Eucheuma denticulatum*, respectively, while cold-water species comprising both haploid and diploid *Chondrus crispus/Gigartina stellate* species produce κ-carrageenan and a mixture of κ-carrageenan and λ-carrageenan, respectively [85,89,98,99]. Carrageenan types form different gels at room temperature, namely κ-carrageenan forms strong and brittle gels, ι-carrageenan forms soft and elastic gels, while λ-carrageenan cannot form gels [93,96,99]. κ-carrageenan isolated from *Hypnea musciformis* red algae exhibited neuroprotective activity in 6-hydroxydopamine-induced neurotoxicity on SH-SY5Y cells by modulating mitochondria transmembrane potential and reducing caspase-3 activity [100].

Fucoidan comprises a complex family of natural water-soluble sulfated polysaccharides [69,95,101–103] containing long type I and type II branched chains. Type I chains contain repeating (1,3)-linked α-L-fucopyranose residues, while type II chains contain alternating (1,3)- and (1,4)-linked α-L-fucopyranose residues. Additionally, these compounds also consist of sulfated galactofucans with backbones built of (1,6)-β-D-galacto- and/or (1, 2)-β-D-mannopyranosyl units and other monosaccharides, including uronic acid, xylose, rhamnose, glucose, arabinose, and xylose [69,95,101,102,104]. Fucoidans are mainly isolated from the cell wall and mucous matrix of various species of brown algae, such as mozuku, kombu, limu moui, bladderwrack, and wakame [69,101,102]. Generally, seaweed species, geographic location, and extraction season and procedures directly influence the molecular weight, monosaccharide composition, and sulfate content and position [95,101,105]. Fucoidan has received considerable scientific interest for its neuroprotection activities. In this regard, Ecklonia cava-extracted fucoidan showed significant antioxidant activities on hydrogen peroxide-induced cytotoxicity in PC-12 and MCIXC cells and neuron-protective effects comparable to vitamin C, by regulating mitochondrial function and acetylcholinesterase inhibition [106]. Similarly, the effects induced by the combination of non-invasive low intensity pulsed electric field and fucoidan against hydrogen peroxide-induced neuronal damage were investigated on the motor neuron-like cell line NSC-34, showing improved results and neuroprotective potential [107]. Furthermore, one study proved the protective activity of *Sargassum hemiphyllum*-extracted fucoidan against 6-hydroxydopamine-induced apoptosis on SH-SY5Y cells [108]. One group investigated the neuroprotective effects of five distinct fucoidan types prepared from *Fucus vesiculosus* and *Undaria pinnatifida* against amyloid-β aggregation and cytotoxicity. They demonstrated a wide range of neuroprotective activities that may have the potential to alter amyloid-β neurotoxicity in AD [109]. Additionally, *Laminaria japonica*-extracted fucoidan was investigated for its protective effects on the dopamine system and mitochondrial function of dopaminergic neurons in the rotenone-induced PD rat model. Results showed a significantly reversed nigral dopaminergic neuron and striatal dopaminergic fiber loss, reduced mitochondrial respiratory function as detected by the mitochondrial oxygen consumption, and ameliorated behavioral deficits [110]. Moreover, fucoidan has proved its potential in the treatment of transient global cerebral ischemia in gerbil models by relieving the acceleration and exacerbation of ischemic brain injury through the attenuation of oxidative damage and glial cell activation [111,112].

Laminarin or laminaran is a biodegradable and non-toxic linear polysaccharide consisting of β-D-glucans linked by (1,3) and (1,6) glycosidic bonds at different ratios. It is extracted from the cell wall of brown seaweeds, such as Laminariaceae, the original source, but also from *Laminaria, Saccharina*, or *Eisenia* species [67,95]. Laminarin has been investigated for its neuroprotective effects in the Cornu Ammonis 1 field of the hippocampus, which is highly vulnerable to ischemia-reperfusion injury, following transient forebrain ischemia in gerbils using histopathological samples. While pretreatment with 10 mg/kg failed to protect neurons, 50 or 100 mg/kg proved to be efficient as a preventive strategy against injuries following cerebral ischemic insults by attenuating reactive gliosis and reducing pro-inflammatory microglia [113]. While such a dose is relatively high, further studies that focus on elucidating the mechanisms responsible for the neuroprotective action could lead to a decrease in the necessary dose and an enhanced activity.

4. Marine Glycosaminoglycans for Neuroprotection

Chemically, glycosaminoglycans are long linear heteropolysaccharides consisting of repeating disaccharide units comprising an amino sugar, either N-acetylgalactosamine or N-acetylglucosamine, and uronic acid, either glucuronate or iduronate [114–116]. Additionally, sulfate and hydroxyl groups can be present, imparting a strong negative charge and an extended conformation [114]. Excepting hyaluronic acid, glycosaminoglycan chains form proteoglycans by covalently binding to polypeptides as core proteins [114,117]. Although most commercial glycosaminoglycans are extracted from terrestrial animals, marine glycosaminoglycans have achieved a great scientific interest as they are different in terms of molecular weight and sulfation and, consequently, biological activity [118]. Hyaluronic acid (HA), chondroitin sulfate (CS), and heparin and heparan sulfate (HS) (Table 2, Figure 2) are the most physiologically important glycosaminoglycans involved in neuroprotective activities that can be extracted from marine sources.

Table 2. The sources of the main marine-derived glycosaminoglycans.

Biocompound	Marine Sources
Hyaluronic acid	marine bivalves (*Mytilus galloprovincialis* and *Amussium pleuronectus*), stingray (*Aetobatus narinari*), mussels, codfish bones, tuna eyeballs, and shark fins
Chondroitin sulfate	blackmouth catshark (*Galeus melastomus*), corb (*Sciaena umbra*), and shark and fish cartilage
Heparin and heparan sulfate	mollusks (bivalves, gastropods, and cephalopods species), sea cucumbers, shrimp heads (*Litopenaeus vannamei* and *Penaeus brasiliensis*), clams (*Anomalocardia brasiliana, Tivela mactroides, Donax striatus*, and *Tapes phlippinarum*), crabs (*Goniopsis cruentata* and *Ucides cordatus*), scallop (*Nodipecten nodosus*), ascidian (*Styela plicata*), sand dollar (*Mellita quinquisperforata*), and cockle (*Cerastoderma edule*)

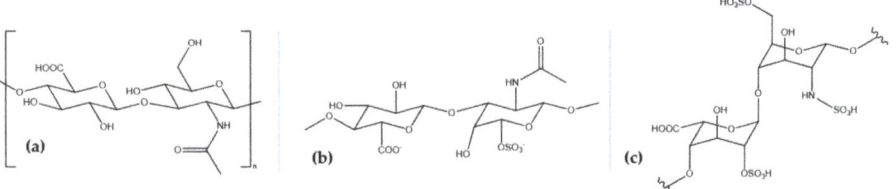

Figure 2. The structure of the main marine-derived glycosaminoglycans: (a) hyaluronic acid; (b) chondroitin sulfate; (c) heparin and heparan sulfate.

HA, also known as hyaluronan, is a natural linear, anionic, non-sulfated polysaccharide produced through the polymerization of D-glucuronic acid and N-acetyl-D-glucosamine linked by alternating glucuronidic β-(1,3) or β-(1,4) bonds, activated by the hyaluronan synthase enzyme [89,116,119–124]. It provides the backbone for specifically binding domains in the aggregating proteoglycan aggrecan [119,122]. HA is a naturally occurring biopolymer with biocompatible, biodegradable, and viscoelastic properties and a molecular weight ranging from 50 kDa to 2 million kDa [89,123]. As the last decade has witnessed a growing interest in isolating HA from marine organisms, several groups have reported the extraction of low molecular weight HA from the marine bivalves *Mytilus galloprovincialis* and *Amussium pleuronectus* and high molecular weight HA from stingray (*Aetobatus narinari*) liver [125]. Other marine sources include mussels, codfish bones, tuna eyeballs, and shark fins [126]. HA has been investigated for its neuroprotective potential in spinal cord injuries. Specifically, a HA/methylcellulose hydrogel was injected into a syringomyelia rat model, showing improved tissue and functional responses and reduced lipopolysaccharide-mediated microglial activation in vitro [127]. Moreover, this type of hydrogel has been modified with an anti-inflammatory peptide and a brain-derived neurotrophic factor, which significantly enhanced the proliferation of PC12 cells and the recovery in both neurological function and nerve tissue morphology in rat models by regulating inflammatory cytokine levels and improving axonal regeneration [128]. Additionally, HA has also proved its efficiency in stroke management, as neuroglobin-loaded sodium hyaluronate nanoparticles have been intravenously introduced in rat models and reached damaged cerebral parenchyma at early stages [129].

CS is a linear and sulfated polysaccharide consisting of repeating disaccharide units of β-(1,4)-D-glucuronic acid and β-(1,3)-N-acetylgalactosamine, which are usually covalently linked to proteins, forming proteoglycans [130–132]. Furthermore, depending on the position of the sulfate group on the polysaccharide backbone, CS can be classified into CS-A (carbon 4), CS-C (carbon 6), CS-E (both carbon 4 and 6), CS-D (position 6 of N-acetylgalactosamine and position 4 of D-glucuronic acid), and CS-B (position 4 of N-acetylgalactosamine and position 2 of D-glucuronic acid) [130,133]. Their versatility has led to a broad range of biological activities and various therapeutic, pharmacological, and nutraceutical applications [134]. Moreover, depending on the sources, either terrestrial or marine, CS contains various chain lengths and oversulfated disaccharides at different relative concentrations, i.e., shark, CS-D, dogfish, CS-A and CS-D, squid and salmon, CS-E, and ray, CS-A and CS-C [133]. Specifically, studies have reported the isolation of CS from the blackmouth catshark (*Galeus melastomus*) [118], corb (*Sciaena umbra*) skin [135], and various shark and other fish cartilage [136]. Experimental researches have indicated the benefits of CS in the therapy of neurodegenerative diseases [137], with one study reporting the neuroprotective effects of CS against advanced glycation end products-induced toxicity, which has been linked to amyloid-β aggregation, oxidative stress, and inflammation [138]. Moreover, low molecular weight CS and selenium-CS nanoparticles have been shown to protect SH-SY5Y cells by inhibiting amyloid-β aggregation, decreasing reactive oxygen species and malondialdehyde levels, and increasing glutathione peroxidase levels [139,140].

Heparin and HS are the most structurally complex glycosaminoglycans, consisting of identical repeating disaccharide units of hexuronic acid, which can be either β-D-glucuronic acid or its C-5 differential isomer, α-L-iduronic acid, and N-acetylgalactosamine through 1,4 linkages. The 2-O position of the hexuronic acid can be sulfated and the 3-O and 6-O positions of the glucosamine can be replaced by an O-sulfo group. The probability of 6-O substitution is greater than 3-O, and the amino group can be sulfonated, acetylated, or unmodified. Heparin and HS have similar structures, but differ in terms of monomer proportion, i.e., heparin has a large proportion of iduronic acid, while HS mainly consists of glucuronic acid. Additionally, heparin has an average of 2.7 sulfated groups compared to 1 in HS, but a lower molecular weight, 12 kDa compared to 30 kDa. Moreover, while heparin is the most negatively charged macromolecule of the human body and, therefore, the most acidic one, HS is characterized by a higher structural heterogeneity [141,142]. The arrangement of the sulfate groups in short segments of the chains produces binding sites for protein ligands to form proteoglycans through O-ether linkages [143–145]. Marine animals are evolutionarily secluded from terrestrial mammals, and they represent an important source of heparin and HS extraction, as there is a lower risk of microorganism contamination. Thus, marine mollusks, such as bivalves, gastropods, and cephalopods species, sea cucumbers [146], shrimp heads (*Litopenaeus vannamei* and *Penaeus brasiliensis*), clams (*Anomalocardia brasiliana*, *Tivela mactroides*, *Donax striatus*, and *Tapes phlippinarum*), crabs (*Goniopsis cruentata* and *Ucides cordatus*), scallop (*Nodipecten nodosus*), ascidian (*Styela plicata*), sand dollar (*Mellita quinquisperforata*) [147], and cockle (*Cerastoderma edule*) [148] represent great sources of heparin and HS. One study investigated the effects of heparin, heparinase III, chondroitinase, hyaluronic acid, and an MMP-2/9 inhibitor together with amyloid-β oligomers on cortical and hippocampal populations generated from human-induced pluripotent stem cell-derived neural spheroids. Results showed that heparin administration reduces amyloid-β-related neural cell death [149]. Furthermore, heparin administration in gerbils proved that pre-treatment considerably reduces neuronal cell apoptosis and expression of tumor necrosis factor-α and interleukin-1β, thus exerting neuroprotective effects against cerebral ischemia/reperfusion injury [150]. Additionally, HS is a promising therapeutic strategy to protect and repair the brain after stroke, favoring functional recovery [151].

5. Marine Glycoproteins for Neuroprotection

Lectins are clusters of oligomeric carbohydrate-binding glycoproteins ubiquitously found in animals, plants, and microorganisms. The "lectin" term is derived from the "legere" Latin word, which means "to select"; precisely, they have a highly specific carbohydrate recognition domain, which offers them the capacity to specifically and reversibly bind to sugar moieties [152–156]. Lectins are a diversified group of proteins of nonimmune origin with many biological roles, including aggregation of animal cells, as they are often referred to as "agglutins", mediation of cell–cell interactions, homeostatic regulation, and immune recognition of foreign carbohydrates [152,154,155]. Depending on their amino acid sequence and biochemical actions, lectins can be classified in several families. Specifically, lectins in fish include C-type lectins, galectins, pentraxins, X-type lectins/intelectins, calnexin, and calreticulin, which can be found in other animals, and F-type lectins, rhamnose-binding lectins, and pufflectins, which have been discovered in fish. They fulfill different biological roles, such as pathogen recognition and opsonization, complement activation, immune function regulation, or they act as antifreeze proteins or prevent polyspermy during fertilization [155]. So far, lectins have been isolated from a variety of marine animals, such as sponges (*Aplysina lactuca*, *Cliona varians*, *Suberites domuncula*, *Axinella corrugata*, and *Chondrilla caribensis*), annelids (*Cinachyrella apion*, *Chaetopterus variopedatus* and *Serpula vermicularis*), mollusks (*Aplysia dactylomela*, *Mytilus galloprovincialis*, *Argopecten irradians*, *Ruditapes philippinarum*, *Madiolus modiolus*, and *Crenomytilus grayanus*), arthropods (*Tachypleus tridentatus* and *Penaeus monodon*), sea cucumbers (*Holothuria scabra*, *Holothuria grisea*, and *Cucumaria echinata*), ascidians (*Didemnum ternatanum*), amphioxus (*Branchiostoma belcheri* and *Branchiostoma japonicum*), and fish (*Aristichtys nobilis*, *Silurus asotus*, *Oncorhynchus tshawytscha*, *Epinephelus coioides*, *Oncorhynchus mykiss*, *Rachycentron canadum*, and *Paralichthys olivaceus*) [157,158]. As they have the ability to modulate molecular targets in the central nervous system, lectins might be involved in processes associated with neuroplasticity, neurobehavioral effects, and neuroprotection [159]. Therefore, galectin-3, a β-galactoside-binding lectin, could modulate the innate immunity and induce a therapeutic shift in microglia polarization, significantly reducing the infarct size, in the context of ischemic injury [160]. Similarly, pentraxin-3, an angiogenesis key regulator, has demonstrated its potential and clinical relevance by providing sustained long-term neurovascular repair after stroke and reducing neuronal loss [161].

6. Marine Lipids and Glycolipids for Neuroprotection

Lipids are responsible for various complex and physiological roles, including cell membrane formation, cell transport, energy storage, signaling, and transmembrane protein modulation. Their composition in the brain depends on age, sex, neuron activity, stress, and trauma, and variations in their concentration, organization, and metabolism might consequently lead to neurological and/or mental disorders [162]. In the brain, the most abundantly found organic compounds are polyunsaturated fatty acids, which are further classified into ω-6 and ω-3 polyunsaturated fatty acids, derived from linoleic acid and α-linolenic acid, respectively [162,163]. While they were generally ignored for more than 40 years, polyunsaturated fatty acids are essential for normal brain development and function [162–166]. ω-3 fatty acids play fundamentally important biological roles, including neurotransmission, signal transduction, receptor binding, and eicosanoid synthesis, and aid in synaptic plasticity and neuroprotection [165,166]. A lack of ω-3 fatty acids has been linked to a chronic pro-inflammatory state in the brain that further leads to dementia and an increased risk of cerebral ischemia [167].

Examples of fatty acids include docosahexaenoic acid, eicosapentaenoic acid, α-linolenic acid, arachidonic acid, linolenic acid, and oleic acid (Table 3, Figure 3) [168]. Fish oils, especially cod liver oil from Atlantic cod (*Gadus Morrhua* L.), are the main source of ω-3 fatty acids [169]. Additionally, microalgae are emerging as a new source for extraction in order to sustain the needs of the population. Due to their increased bioactivity, docosahexaenoic acid, and eicosapentaenoic acid are the most nutritionally significant fatty acids produced [170].

Table 3. The sources of the main polyunsaturated fatty acids obtained from marine sources.

Biocompound	Marine Sources
docosahexaenoic acid	
eicosapentaenoic acid	
α-linolenic acid	fish oils, marine algae, sea cucumber, microalgae
arachidonic acid	
linoleic acid	
oleic acid	

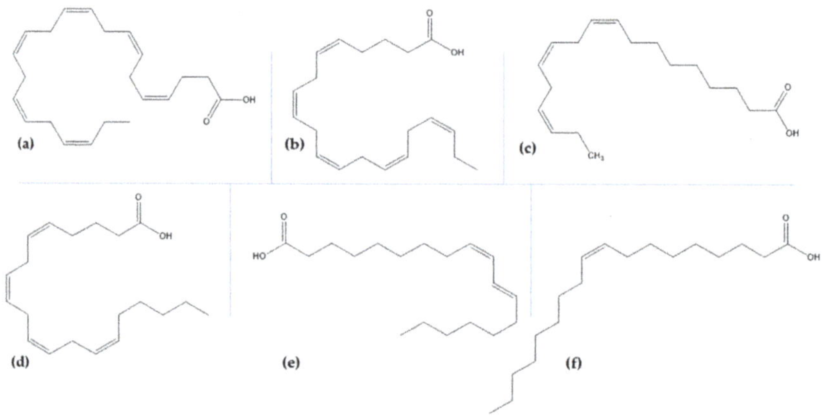

Figure 3. The structure of the main polyunsaturated fatty acids obtained from marine sources: (**a**) docosahexaenoic acid; (**b**) eicosapentaenoic acid; (**c**) α-linolenic acid; (**d**) arachidonic acid; (**e**) linoleic acid; (**f**) oleic acid.

As some studies reported the beneficial effects of some polyunsaturated fatty acids in AD by reducing amyloid-β toxicity through enhancing its degradation and clearance, one group investigated the interactions of fatty acids docosahexaenoic acid, eicosatetraenoic acid, α-linolenic acid, arachidonic acid, linoleic acid, and oleic acid with amyloid-β peptides. Results showed that all the fatty acids tested have anti-aggregation properties by preventing amyloid-β40 and amyloid-β42 fibrillogenesis, thus providing a novel direction for developing a therapy for AD [171]. Furthermore, docosahexaenoic acid has been shown to play a crucial role in neurogenesis, antinociceptive effects, anti-apoptotic effects, synaptic plasticity, Ca^{2+} homeostasis in brain diseases, and nigrostriatal activity functioning, with a high intake of docosahexaenoic acid-containing foods being linked with a lower risk of AD and other brain disorders [172]. In this regard, one study showed that the administration of docosahexaenoic acid-enriched phosphatidylcholine and docosahexaenoic acid-enriched phosphatidylserine in AD SAMP8 mice models improved the metabolic disorders and cognitive deficits by ameliorating amyloid-β pathology, mitochondrial damage, neuroinflammation, and neurotrophic factors and oxidative stress, respectively. The molecular mechanisms responsible have been found to be closely related to the phospholipid polar groups [173]. Moreover, the effects of docosahexaenoic acid and eicosapentaenoic acid, either alone or in combinations of 1:1, 1:2 and 2:1, as found in sea seals, sea algae, and fish oil, on cellular models of AD have been investigated. Results demonstrated that both fatty acids attenuate neuron apoptosis and improve cell viability with synergistic anti-inflammatory effects in the AD model; additionally, pure eicosapentaenoic acid is more effective against oxidative stress, while pure docosahexaenoic acid better improves neurotrophic systems [174]. Furthermore, eicosapentaenoic acid-enriched phospholipids extracted from the sea cucumber (*Cucumaria frondosa*) improved MPTP-induced PD in mice by suppressing oxidative stress and apoptosis and alleviating the loss of dopaminergic neurons via mitochondria-mediated and mitogen-activated protein kinase pathways [175].

Glycolipids comprise a large class of natural compounds consisting of a glycosidic fragment linked to a lipid molecule. Although highly structurally variable, glycolipids can be classified into three main categories, namely glycosphingolipids, glycoglycerolipids, and atypical glycolipids [176].

Chemically, glycosphingolipids comprise sphingosine and fatty acid residues, which are linked to an amide in the ceramide and contain no phosphate groups. Furthermore, a carbohydrate links through a β-glycosidic bond to the primary alcohol oxygen atom of the ceramide [177]. Glycosphingolipids represent the building blocks of the outer leaflet of the cell membrane in a wide variety of terrestrial and marine organisms, where they play fundamental physiological roles due to variations in the sugar chains. They are continuously recycled inside lysosomes by glycosidase fragmentation [178,179]. Based on the constituent sugars, glycosphingolipids can be further classified into cerebrosides, ceramide oligohexosides, globosides, and gangliosides. Echinoderms, porifera, and mollusks have been identified as suitable marine sources for glycosphingolipid isolation [179]. One study investigated the protective effects of sea cucumber-derived cerebrosides against amyloid-β-induced cognitive impairment on AD male rat models. Results proved the neuroprotective capacity of the marine-derived glycolipids by ameliorating neuronal damage and suppressing the induced apoptosis [180]. Moreover, gangliosides, a family of glycosphingolipids containing sialic acid linked to an oligoglycosyl backbone, which is further attached to a ceramide base, are highly expressed in vertebrate nervous systems [181]. Additionally, they are widely present in marine echinoderms, such as sea cucumbers, sea urchins, and starfishes, which are found to be different from mammalian glycosphingolipids in terms of their basic sugar moiety and the types and numbers of sialic acids (i.e., mammalian glycosphingolipids contain mainly N-acetyl-neuraminic acid, while echinoderm glycosphingolipids contain N-acetyl-neuraminic acid, N-glycolylneuraminic acid, and sulfated N-glycolylneuraminic acid). One study reported the neuroprotective effects of the sea urchin *Strongylocentrotus nudus*-isolated glycosphingolipids on AD models of Ab25-35-induced PC12 cells and SAMP8 mice as in vitro and in vivo models. The main mechanisms involve inhibition of synaptic loss through synaptophysin and GAP-43 expression and mediation of mitochondrial apoptosis, which is directly related to the neurofibrillary pathology [182].

Furthermore, glycoglycerolipids are ubiquitously found in the chloroplasts of eukaryotic algae, but also in cyanobacteria or other higher plants. Their basic structure involves a 1,2-diacyl-sn-glycerol moiety and mono- or oligosaccharides attached at the sn-3 position of the glycerol backbone. The three major types of glycoglycerolipids include monogalactosyldiacylglycerol (1,2-diacyl-3-O-(β-D-galactopyranosyl)-sn-glycerol), digalactosyldiacylglycerol 1,2-diacyl-3-O-(α-D-galactopyranosyl-(1′,6)-O-β-D-galactopyranosyl)-sn-glycerol), and sulfoquinovosyldiacylglycerol (1,2-diacyl-3-O-(6-deoxy-6-sulfo-α-D-glucopyranosyl)-sn-glycerol) [179,183].

Marine microbial-derived glycolipids have been intensively studied since they are widely produced by a broad spectrum of bacteria extracted from different marine matrices, including animals, e.g., Annelida, *Pteroides spinosum*, or fish gut, and contaminated soils [184]. Furthermore, microalgae have become a promising lipid source due to their lipid accumulation mechanisms triggered by various stress conditions, such as limited nutrients or damaging physical factors [185]. Generally, they produce a great variety of lipids, including polar lipids, neutral lipids, wax esters, hydrocarbons, or sterols [186].

7. Marine Pigments for Neuroprotection

Pigments are molecular structures capable of absorbing specific wavelengths of light and reflecting the rest of the visible spectrum. Moreover, microbial pigments possess additional chemical component mixtures that have complex biological activities, such as antimicrobial, anticancer, and immunomodulation. Thus, recent years have witnessed a tremendous increase in the study of terrestrial and marine microbial pigments [187–191]. The production of pigments by marine bacteria is presumably mediated by the quorum-sensing mechanism [188]. Most common types of pigment compounds from marine microorganisms include carotenoids, polyunsaturated hydrocarbons with 30, 40, or 50 carbon atoms in one molecule, melanins, polyphenolic pigments obtained through hydroxylation, oxidation, and polymerization reactions of phenolic compounds, phenazines, tricyclic, redox-active, and small nitrogen-containing heterocyclic aromatic compounds, prodiginines, aromatic chemical compounds with pyrrolyl dipyrromethene core structures, quinones, compounds containing aromatic ring structures with yellow-to-red color hues, tambjamines, alkaloid compounds with yellow color hues, and violacein, indole-pigmented compounds derived from the metabolism of tryptophan [188].

Carotenoids, the most abundant naturally occurring pigments, have received a great scientific interest owing to their potentially beneficial uses in healthcare, pharmaceuticals, and biotechnologies [39,192]. Since the structural elucidation of β-carotene in 1930, about 750 natural carotenoids have been described, among which more than 250 are of marine origin [193]. Carotenoids are generally divided into carotenes, strict hydrocarbon carotenoids with no substituent in their structures, and xanthophylls, oxygen-containing molecules [194]. Among them, the most common carotenoids produced by marine microorganisms, e.g., microalgae, bacteria, archaea, fungi, and fungi-like protists, are β-carotene, astaxanthin, canthaxanthin, β-cryptoxanthin, diadinoxanthin, dinoxanthin, echinenone, fucoxanthin, lycopene, lutein, zeaxanthin, violaxanthin, and rare carotenoids, including bacterioruberin, myxol, salinixanthin, saproxanthin, sioxanthin, and siphonaxanthin. Their extraction is performed by controlling and optimizing the conditions of growth, using fast and low cost techniques [192–194].

On the one hand, lycopene is a biocompound that has been widely researched owing to its beneficial effects in the central nervous system. One study proved its potential to attenuate oxidative stress and reduce tert-butyl hydroperoxide-induced cell apoptosis as key factors in the pathogenesis of AD. Lycopene administration led to improved cell viability and neuron morphology, increased GSH/GSSG levels, restored mitochondrial membrane potential, and decreased reactive oxygen species [195]. Similarly, intragastric pretreatment resulted in reduced inflammatory cytokine levels and reversed amyloid-β-induced up-regulation of TLR4 and NF-κB p65 mRNA and protein expressions at the choroid plexus, thereby diminishing amyloid-β deposition in the hippocampus [196]. Additionally, the administration of lycopene has led to alleviated cognition impairment and oxidative stress by decreasing malondialdehyde and 8-hydroxy-2′-deoxyguanosine levels and increasing glutathione level and superoxide dismutase activity in aluminum chloride-induced hippocampal lesions in rat models. These mechanisms have proved to subsequently prevent neuroinflammation and apoptosis [197]. Furthermore, lycopene exhibited neuroprotective effects in MPTP-treated PD mice models by increasing dopamine levels and decreasing oxidative stress levels [198]. Lycopene has also proved to be useful in spinal cord ischemia/reperfusion injury rat models, by improving neurological function recovery and suppressing neuronal death and neuroinflammation [199] and hyperlipidemia-induced cerebral vessel injury prevention by decreasing astrocytes activation and inflammatory cytokine production [200].

On the other hand, astaxanthin, a xanthophyll carotenoid compound, has proved its neuroprotective potential through the inhibition of lipopolysaccharide-induced neuroinflammation, amyloidogenesis, and oxidant activity in mice models [201] and the prevention of hippocampal insulin resistance and AD complications in Wistar rats [202] and brain damage in offspring exposed to prenatal epilepsy seizures [203]. Additionally, astaxanthin and fucoxanthin have also been investigated for their neuroprotective potential against amyloid-β-mediated toxicity in pheochromocytoma neuronal cells. Results demonstrated multi-neuroprotective effects but suggested a higher potential of fucoxanthin as a potential therapeutic strategy [204]. Crocin has also been administered for the therapy of AD and PD, with results proving the potential to treat neurodegeneration [205–207]. Additionally, the potential of β-carotene for the treatment of acute spinal cord injury has been investigated, and results showed a reduced progression of secondary injury events through the prevention of the nuclear factor–κB pathway [208].

8. Conclusions

As natural products are preferred for the discovery and development of drug molecules for the treatment of various human diseases, there have been considerable advancements in the pharmaceutical biocompound industry. Although terrestrial organisms are currently the main source, the marine environment has received significant scientific interest due to its biodiversity, abundancy, and the biological potential of the derived biocompounds. Additionally, their structural and chemical properties are not generally found in terrestrial products, exhibiting considerable bioactivity ten times higher than terrestrial-sourced molecules. Marine biocompounds are of animal, plant, and microorganism origin, each type providing a plethora of compounds, including carbohydrates, polyphenols, peptides, proteins, pigments, and essential fatty acids, that exhibit antioxidant, anti-thrombotic, anti-coagulant, anti-inflammatory, anti-proliferative, anti-hypertensive, anti-diabetic, and cardio-protection properties. Moreover, marine biocompounds have proved their neuroprotective effects through various research studies, mainly aiming at the prevention of neurodegeneration and the reduction of oxidative stress in the central nervous system. However, the field of marine-sourced neuroprotective compounds is still in its infancy, requiring further discoveries and investigations.

Author Contributions: A.F.B., C.C., A.M.G. have participated in review writing and revision. All authors have read and agreed to the published version of the manuscript.

Funding: This research received no external funding.

Acknowledgments: This research has no acknowledgment.

Conflicts of Interest: The authors declare no conflict of interest.

References

1. Gong, H.; Luo, Z.; Chen, W.; Feng, Z.-P.; Wang, G.-L.; Sun, H.-S. Marine Compound Xyloketal B as a Potential Drug Development Target for Neuroprotection. *Marine Drugs* **2018**, *16*, 516. [CrossRef] [PubMed]
2. Amer, M.S.; Barakat, K.M.; Hassanein, A.E.A. Phthalate derivatives from marine Penicillium decumbens and its synergetic effect against sepsis bacteria. *Biointerface Res. Appl. Chem.* **2019**, *9*, 4070–4076.
3. Khalifa, S.A.M.; Elias, N.; Farag, M.A.; Chen, L.; Saeed, A.; Hegazy, M.-E.F.; Moustafa, M.S.; Abd El-Wahed, A.; Al-Mousawi, S.M.; Musharraf, S.G.; et al. Marine Natural Products: A Source of Novel Anticancer Drugs. *Mar. Drugs* **2019**, *17*, 491. [CrossRef] [PubMed]
4. Malve, H. Exploring the ocean for new drug developments: Marine pharmacology. *J. Pharm. Bioallied Sci.* **2016**, *8*, 83–91. [CrossRef]
5. Khan, R.A. Natural products chemistry: The emerging trends and prospective goals. *Saudi Pharm. J.* **2018**, *26*, 739–753. [CrossRef]

6. Dias-Souza, M.V.; Dias, C.G.; Ferreira-Marçal, P.H. Interactions of natural products and antimicrobial drugs: Investigations of a dark matter in chemistry. *Biointerface Res. Appl. Chem.* **2018**, *8*, 3259–3264.
7. Manciu, F.S.; Ciubuc, J.D.; Ochoa, K.; Dacha, P.; Subedi, M.; Guerrero, J.; Eastman, M.; Hodges, D.R.; Bennet, K.E. Comparative spectroscopic analysis of nordihydroguaiaretic acid and related natural products to inhibition of calcium oxalate calculi. *Biointerface Res. Appl. Chem.* **2019**, *9*, 3942–3948.
8. Moss, N.A.; Leao, T.; Glukhov, E.; Gerwick, L.; Gerwick, W.H. Chapter One—Collection, Culturing, and Genome Analyses of Tropical Marine Filamentous Benthic Cyanobacteria. In *Methods in Enzymology*; Moore, B.S., Ed.; Academic Press: Cambridge, MA, USA, 2018; Volume 604, pp. 3–43.
9. Hamed, I.; Özogul, F.; Özogul, Y.; Regenstein, J.M. Marine Bioactive Compounds and Their Health Benefits: A Review. *Compr. Rev. Food Sci. Food Saf.* **2015**, *14*, 446–465. [CrossRef]
10. Barbosa, M.; Valentão, P.; Andrade, P. Bioactive Compounds from Macroalgae in the New Millennium: Implications for Neurodegenerative Diseases. *Mar. Drugs* **2014**, *12*, 4934–4972. [CrossRef]
11. Figuerola, B.; Avila, C. The Phylum Bryozoa as a Promising Source of Anticancer Drugs. *Mar. Drugs* **2019**, *17*, 477. [CrossRef]
12. Kosanic, M.; Rankovic, B.; Stanojkovic, T. Evaluation of antioxidant, antimicrobial and anticancer effects of three selected marine macroalgae. *Rom. Biotechnol. Lett.* **2018**, *23*, 13804–13813.
13. Sirakov, I.; Velichkova, K.; Rusenova, N.; Dinev, T. In vitro test of inhibition effect of extracts from three seaweed species distributed at Black sea on different pathogens potentially dangerous for aquaponics. *Rom. Biotechnol. Lett.* **2019**, *24*, 176–183. [CrossRef]
14. Carson, M.A.; Clarke, S.A. Bioactive Compounds from Marine Organisms: Potential for Bone Growth and Healing. *Mar. drugs* **2018**, *16*, 340. [CrossRef] [PubMed]
15. Martins, A.; Vieira, H.; Gaspar, H.; Santos, S. Marketed Marine Natural Products in the Pharmaceutical and Cosmeceutical Industries: Tips for Success. *Mar. Drugs* **2014**, *12*, 1066–1101. [CrossRef] [PubMed]
16. Kirk Cochran, J. Biological Oceanography. In *Reference Module in Earth Systems and Environmental Sciences*; Elsevier: Amsterdam, The Netherlands, 2014. [CrossRef]
17. Blunt, J.W.; Carroll, A.R.; Copp, B.R.; Davis, R.A.; Keyzers, R.A.; Prinsep, M.R. Marine natural products. *Nat. Prod. Rep.* **2018**, *35*, 8–53. [CrossRef] [PubMed]
18. Suleria, H.A.R.; Gobe, G.; Masci, P.; Osborne, S.A. Marine bioactive compounds and health promoting perspectives; innovation pathways for drug discovery. *Trends Food Sci. Technol.* **2016**, *50*, 44–55. [CrossRef]
19. Gan, L.; Cookson, M.R.; Petrucelli, L.; La Spada, A.R. Converging pathways in neurodegeneration, from genetics to mechanisms. *Nat. Neurosci.* **2018**, *21*, 1300–1309. [CrossRef]
20. Farooqui, A.A. Chapter 1—Classification and Molecular Aspects of Neurotraumatic Diseases: Similarities and Differences With Neurodegenerative and Neuropsychiatric Diseases. In *Ischemic and Traumatic Brain and Spinal Cord Injuries*; Farooqui, A.A., Ed.; Academic Press: Cambridge, MA, USA, 2018; pp. 1–40. [CrossRef]
21. Lindholm, D.; Hyrskyluoto, A.; Bruelle, C.; Putkonen, N.; Korhonen, L. Proteasome Role in Neurodegeneration. In *Reference Module in Biomedical Sciences*; Elsevier: Amsterdam, The Netherlands, 2015. [CrossRef]
22. Fan, J.; Dawson, T.M.; Dawson, V.L. Cell Death Mechanisms of Neurodegeneration. In *Neurodegenerative Diseases: Pathology, Mechanisms, and Potential Therapeutic Targets*; Beart, P., Robinson, M., Rattray, M., Maragakis, N.J., Eds.; Springer International Publishing: Berlin/Heidelberg, Germany, 2017; pp. 403–425. [CrossRef]
23. Liu, Y.; Hsu, S.-H. Biomaterials and neural regeneration. *Neural Regen. Res.* **2020**, *15*, 1243–1244.
24. Madore, C.; Yin, Z.; Leibowitz, J.; Butovsky, O. Microglia, Lifestyle Stress, and Neurodegeneration. *Immunity* **2020**, *52*, 222–240. [CrossRef]
25. Sánchez-López, E.; Marina, M.L. Chapter 20—Neuroscience Applications of Capillary Electrophoretic Methods. In *Capillary Electromigration Separation Methods*; Poole, C.F., Ed.; Elsevier: Amsterdam, The Netherlands, 2018; pp. 481–510. [CrossRef]
26. Sardoiwala, M.N.; Kaundal, B.; Roy Choudhury, S. Chapter 37—Development of Engineered Nanoparticles Expediting Diagnostic and Therapeutic Applications Across Blood–Brain Barrier. In *Handbook of Nanomaterials for Industrial Applications*; Hussain, C.M., Ed.; Elsevier: Amsterdam, The Netherlands, 2018; pp. 696–709. [CrossRef]

27. Brahmachari, G. Chapter 1—Discovery and development of anti-inflammatory agents from natural products: An overview. In *Discovery and Development of Anti-Inflammatory Agents from Natural Products*, Brahmachari, G., Ed.; Elsevier: Amsterdam, The Netherlands, 2019; pp. 1–6. [CrossRef]
28. Huang, M.; Gu, X.; Gao, X. 13—Nanotherapeutic strategies for the treatment of neurodegenerative diseases. In *Brain Targeted Drug Delivery System*; Gao, H., Gao, X., Eds.; Academic Press: Cambridge, MA, USA, 2019; pp. 321–356. [CrossRef]
29. Anitha, A.; Thanseem, I.; Vasu, M.M.; Viswambharan, V.; Poovathinal, S.A. Chapter Three—Telomeres in neurological disorders. In *Advances in Clinical Chemistry*; Makowski, G.S., Ed.; Elsevier: Amsterdam, The Netherlands, 2019; Volume 90, pp. 81–132.
30. Magalingam, K.B.; Radhakrishnan, A.; Ping, N.S.; Haleagrahara, N. Current Concepts of Neurodegenerative Mechanisms in Alzheimer's Disease. *BioMed. Res. Int.* **2018**, *2018*, 3740461. [CrossRef]
31. Sharma, N. Chapter 142—Parkinson Disease. In *Essentials of Physical Medicine and Rehabilitation*, 4th ed.; Frontera, W.R., Silver, J.K., Rizzo, T.D., Eds.; Elsevier: Philadelphia, PA, USA, 2020; pp. 806–810. [CrossRef]
32. Niethammer, M.; Eidelberg, D. Chapter Five—Network Imaging in Parkinsonian and Other Movement Disorders: Network Dysfunction and Clinical Correlates. In *International Review of Neurobiology*; Politis, M., Ed.; Academic Press: Cambridge, MA, USA, 2019; Volume 144, pp. 143–184.
33. Kim, S.D.; Allen, N.E.; Canning, C.G.; Fung, V.S.C. Chapter 11—Parkinson disease. In *Handbook of Clinical Neurology*; Day, B.L., Lord, S.R., Eds.; Elsevier: Amsterdam, The Netherlands, 2018; Volume 159, pp. 173–193.
34. Gozes, I.; Levine, J. Introduction. In *Neuroprotection in Autism, Schizophrenia and Alzheimer's Disease*; Gozes, I., Levine, J., Eds.; Academic Press: Cambridge, MA, USA, 2020; pp. Xiii–xvii. [CrossRef]
35. Teleanu, R.I.; Gherasim, O.; Gherasim, T.G.; Grumezescu, V.; Grumezescu, A.M.; Teleanu, D.M. Nanomaterial-Based Approaches for Neural Regeneration. *Pharmaceutics* **2019**, *11*, 266. [CrossRef] [PubMed]
36. Gonzalez Nieto, D.; Fernández-Serra, R.; Pérez-Rigueiro, J.; Panetsos, F.; Martinez-Murillo, R.; Guinea, G. Biomaterials to Neuroprotect the Stroke Brain: A Large Opportunity for Narrow Time Windows. *Cells* **2020**, *9*, 1074. [CrossRef] [PubMed]
37. Fernandez-Serra, R.; Gallego, R.; Lozano, P.; Gonzalez-Nieto, D. Hydrogels for neuroprotection and functional rewiring: A new era for brain engineering. *Neural Regen. Res.* **2020**, *15*, 783–789. [PubMed]
38. Wasik, A.; Antkiewicz-Michaluk, L. The mechanism of neuroprotective action of natural compounds. *Pharmacol. Rep.: PR* **2017**, *69*, 851–860. [CrossRef]
39. Teleanu, R.I.; Chircov, C.; Grumezescu, A.M.; Volceanov, A.; Teleanu, D.M. Antioxidant Therapies for Neuroprotection—A Review. *J. Clin. Med.* **2019**, *8*, 1659. [CrossRef]
40. Ruocco, N.; Costantini, S.; Guariniello, S.; Costantini, M. Polysaccharides from the marine environment with pharmacological, cosmeceutical and nutraceutical potential. *Molecules* **2016**, *21*, 551. [CrossRef]
41. Shang, Q.; Jiang, H.; Cai, C.; Hao, J.; Li, G.; Yu, G. Gut microbiota fermentation of marine polysaccharides and its effects on intestinal ecology: An overview. *Carbohydr. Polym.* **2017**, *179*. [CrossRef]
42. Tang, Y.; Cui, Y.; De Agostini, A.; Zhang, L. Chapter Eighteen—Biological mechanisms of glycan- and glycosaminoglycan-based nutraceuticals. In *Progress in Molecular Biology and Translational Science*; Zhang, L., Ed.; Academic Press: Cambridge, MA, USA, 2019; Volume 163, pp. 445–469.
43. Loureiro dos Santos, L.A. Natural Polymeric Biomaterials: Processing and Properties. In *Reference Module in Materials Science and Materials Engineering*; Elsevier: Amsterdam, The Netherlands, 2017. [CrossRef]
44. Deshmukh, K.; Basheer Ahamed, M.; Deshmukh, R.R.; Khadheer Pasha, S.K.; Bhagat, P.R.; Chidambaram, K. 3—Biopolymer Composites With High Dielectric Performance: Interface Engineering. In *Biopolymer Composites in Electronics*; Sadasivuni, K.K., Ponnamma, D., Kim, J., Cabibihan, J.J., AlMaadeed, M.A., Eds.; Elsevier: Amsterdam, The Netherlands, 2017; pp. 27–128. [CrossRef]
45. Cardoso, M.J.; Costa, R.R.; Mano, J.F. Marine Origin Polysaccharides in Drug Delivery Systems. *Mar. drugs* **2016**, *14*, 34. [CrossRef]
46. Rodriguez-Chanfrau, J.E.; Rodriguez-Riera, Z.; Gamiotea-Turro, D. Trimethylchitosan hydrochloride obtained from lobster carapace chitin on a bench scale. *Biointerface Res. Appl. Chem.* **2019**, *9*, 4279–4283.
47. Blanco, A.; Blanco, G. Chapter 4—Carbohydrates. In *Medical Biochemistry*; Blanco, A., Blanco, G., Eds.; Academic Press: Cambridge, MA, USA, 2017; pp. 73–97. [CrossRef]
48. Sánchez-Machado, D.I.; López-Cervantes, J.; Correa-Murrieta, M.A.; Sánchez-Duarte, R.G.; Cruz-Flores, P.; de la Mora-López, G.S. Chapter 4.2—Chitosan. In *Nonvitamin and Nonmineral Nutritional Supplements*; Nabavi, S.M., Silva, A.S., Eds.; Academic Press: Cambridge, MA, USA, 2019; pp. 485–493. [CrossRef]

49. Alamgir, A. *Bioactive Compounds and Pharmaceutical Excipients Derived from Animals, Marine Organisms, Microorganisms, Minerals, Synthesized Compounds, and Pharmaceutical Drugs*; Springer: Berlin/Heidelberg, Germany, 2018; pp. 311–406. [CrossRef]
50. Amanzadi, B.; Mirzaei, E.; Hassanzadeh, G.; Mahdaviani, P.; Boroumand, S.; Abdollahi, M.; Hosseinabdolghaffari, A.; Majidi, R.F. Chitosan-based layered nanofibers loaded with herbal extract as wound-dressing materials on wound model studies. *Biointerface Res. Appl. Chem.* **2019**, *9*, 3979–3986.
51. Das, B.; Patra, S. Chapter 1—Antimicrobials: Meeting the Challenges of Antibiotic Resistance Through Nanotechnology. In *Nanostructures for Antimicrobial Therapy, Ficai, A., Grumezescu, A.M., Eds.*; Elsevier: Amsterdam, The Netherlands, 2017; pp. 1–22. [CrossRef]
52. Faust, H.J.; Guo, Q.; Elisseeff, J.H. Chapter 53—Cartilage Tissue Engineering. In *Principles of Regenerative Medicine*, 3rd ed.; Atala, A., Lanza, R., Mikos, A.G., Nerem, R., Eds.; Academic Press: Cambridge, MA, USA, 2019; pp. 937–952. [CrossRef]
53. Ezzat, H.A.; Hegazy, M.A.; Nada, N.A.; Ibrahim, M.A. Effect of nano metal oxides on the electronic properties of cellulose, chitosan and sodium alginate. *Biointerface Res. Appl. Chem.* **2019**, *9*, 4143–4149.
54. Li, Y.; Ju, D. Chapter 12—The Application, Neurotoxicity, and Related Mechanism of Cationic Polymers. In *Neurotoxicity of Nanomaterials and Nanomedicine*, Jiang, X., Gao, H., Eds.; Academic Press: Cambridge, MA, USA, 2017; pp. 285–329. [CrossRef]
55. Teixeira, M.d.C.; Santini, A.; Souto, E.B. Chapter 8—Delivery of Antimicrobials by Chitosan-Composed Therapeutic Nanostructures. In *Nanostructures for Antimicrobial Therapy*; Ficai, A., Grumezescu, A.M., Eds.; Elsevier: Amsterdam, The Netherlands, 2017; pp. 203–222. [CrossRef]
56. Chen, B.; Li, J.; Borgens, R.B. Neuroprotection by chitosan nanoparticles in oxidative stress-mediated injury. *BMC Res. Notes* **2018**, *11*, 49. [CrossRef] [PubMed]
57. Santos-Moriano, P.; Fernandez-Arrojo, L.; Mengibar, M.; Belmonte-Reche, E.; Peñalver, P.; Acosta, F.N.; Ballesteros, A.O.; Morales, J.C.; Kidibule, P.; Fernandez-Lobato, M.; et al. Enzymatic production of fully deacetylated chitooligosaccharides and their neuroprotective and anti-inflammatory properties. *Biocatal. Biotransformation* **2018**, *36*, 57–67. [CrossRef]
58. He, B.; Wu, F.; Fan, L.; Li, X.H.; Liu, Y.; Liu, Y.J.; Ding, W.J.; Deng, M.; Zhou, Y. Carboxymethylated chitosan protects Schwann cells against hydrogen peroxide-induced apoptosis by inhibiting oxidative stress and mitochondria dependent pathway. *Eur. J. Pharmacol.* **2018**, *825*, 48–56. [CrossRef]
59. Xu, C.; Guan, S.; Wang, B.; Wang, S.; Wang, Y.; Sun, C.; Ma, X.; Liu, T. Synthesis of protocatechuic acid grafted chitosan copolymer: Structure characterization and in vitro neuroprotective potential. *Int. J. Biol. Macromol.* **2018**, *109*, 1–11. [CrossRef]
60. Fachel, F.N.S.; Dal Prá, M.; Azambuja, J.H.; Endres, M.; Bassani, V.L.; Koester, L.S.; Henriques, A.T.; Barschak, A.G.; Teixeira, H.F.; Braganhol, E. Glioprotective Effect of Chitosan-Coated Rosmarinic Acid Nanoemulsions Against Lipopolysaccharide-Induced Inflammation and Oxidative Stress in Rat Astrocyte Primary Cultures. *Cell. Mol. Neurobiol.* **2020**, *40*, 123–139. [CrossRef]
61. Manigandan, V.; Nataraj, J.; Karthik, R.; Manivasagam, T.; Saravanan, R.; Thenmozhi, A.J.; Essa, M.M.; Guillemin, G.J. Low Molecular Weight Sulfated Chitosan: Neuroprotective Effect on Rotenone-Induced In Vitro Parkinson's Disease. *Neurotox. Res.* **2019**, *35*, 505–515. [CrossRef]
62. Md, S.; Alhakamy, N.A.; Aldawsari, H.M.; Asfour, H.Z. Neuroprotective and antioxidant effect of naringenin-loaded nanoparticles for nose-to-brain delivery. *Brain Sci.* **2019**, *9*. [CrossRef]
63. Bhattamisra, S.K.; Shak, A.T.; Xi, L.W.; Safian, N.H.; Choudhury, H.; Lim, W.M.; Shahzad, N.; Alhakamy, N.A.; Anwer, M.K.; Radhakrishnan, A.K.; et al. Nose to brain delivery of rotigotine loaded chitosan nanoparticles in human SH-SY5Y neuroblastoma cells and animal model of Parkinson's disease. *Int. J. Pharm.* **2020**, *579*. [CrossRef]
64. Smriti, O.; Babita, K.; Hina, C. Neuroprotective potential of dimethyl fumarate-loaded polymeric Nanoparticles against multiple sclerosis. *Indian J. Pharm. Sci.* **2019**, *81*, 496–502.
65. Youssef, A.E.H.; Dief, A.E.; El Azhary, N.M.; Abdelmonsif, D.A.; El-fetiany, O.S. LINGO-1 siRNA nanoparticles promote central remyelination in ethidium bromide-induced demyelination in rats. *J. Physiol. Biochem.* **2019**, *75*, 89–99. [CrossRef] [PubMed]
66. Yao, Z.A.; Chen, F.J.; Cui, H.L.; Lin, T.; Guo, N.; Wu, H.G. Efficacy of chitosan and sodium alginate scaffolds for repair of spinal cord injury in rats. *Neural Regen. Res.* **2018**, *13*, 502–509. [PubMed]

67. Zargarzadeh, M.; Amaral, A.J.R.; Custódio, C.A.; Mano, J.F. Biomedical applications of laminarin. *Carbohydr. Polym.* **2020**, *232*, 115774. [CrossRef]
68. Patel, S. 4—Seaweed-Derived Sulfated Polysaccharides: Scopes and Challenges in Implication in Health Care. In *Bioactive Seaweeds for Food Applications*; Qin, Y., Ed.; Academic Press: Cambridge, MA, USA, 2018; pp. 71–93. [CrossRef]
69. Shen, P.; Yin, Z.; Qu, G.; Wang, C. 11—Fucoidan and Its Health Benefits. In *Bioactive Seaweeds for Food Applications*; Qin, Y., Ed.; Academic Press: Cambridge, MA, USA, 2018; pp. 223–238. [CrossRef]
70. Nechifor, R.; Nastuneac, V.; Domingues, V.F.; Figueiredo, S.; De Freitas, O.M.; Delerue-Matos, C.; Lazar, I. The Use of Marine Algae in the Bioremediation of Contaminated Water with Pharmaceutical Products and Persistent Organic Products (POPs). *Rom. Biotechnol. Lett.* **2019**, *24*, 464–471. [CrossRef]
71. Anyanwu, R.C.; Rodriguez, C.; Durrant, A.; Olabi, A.G. Micro-Macroalgae Properties and Applications. In *Reference Module in Materials Science and Materials Engineering*; Elsevier: Amsterdam, The Netherlands, 2018. [CrossRef]
72. Alba, K.; Kontogiorgos, V. Seaweed Polysaccharides (Agar, Alginate Carrageenan). In *Encyclopedia of Food Chemistry*; Melton, L., Shahidi, F., Varelis, P., Eds.; Academic Press: Cambridge, MA, USA, 2019; pp. 240–250. [CrossRef]
73. Alihosseini, F. 10—Plant-based compounds for antimicrobial textiles. In *Antimicrobial Textiles*; Sun, G., Ed.; Woodhead Publishing: Sawton, Cambride, UK, 2016; pp. 155–195. [CrossRef]
74. Tariverdian, T.; Navaei, T.; Milan, P.B.; Samadikuchaksaraei, A.; Mozafari, M. Chapter 16—Functionalized polymers for tissue engineering and regenerative medicines. In *Advanced Functional Polymers for Biomedical Applications*; Mozafari, M., Singh Chauhan, N.P., Eds.; Elsevier: Amsterdam, The Netherlands, 2019; pp. 323–357. [CrossRef]
75. Abhilash, M.; Thomas, D. 15—Biopolymers for Biocomposites and Chemical Sensor Applications. In *Biopolymer Composites in Electronics*; Sadasivuni, K.K., Ponnamma, D., Kim, J., Cabibihan, J.J., AlMaadeed, M.A., Eds.; Elsevier: Amsterdam, The Netherlands, 2017; pp. 405–435. [CrossRef]
76. Abdelghany, A.M.; Meikhail, M.S.; El-Bana, A.A. Microbial activity and swelling behavior of chitosan/polyvinyl alcohol/sodium alginate semi-natural terpolymer interface containing amoxicillin for wound dressing applications. *Biointerface Res. Appl. Chem.* **2019**, *9*, 4368–4373.
77. Takeshita, S.; Oda, T. Chapter Seven—Usefulness of Alginate Lyases Derived from Marine Organisms for the Preparation of Alginate Oligomers with Various Bioactivities. In *Advances in Food and Nutrition Research*; Kim, S.-K., Toldrá, F., Eds.; Academic Press: Cambridge, MA, USA, 2016; Volume 79, pp. 137–160.
78. Azeem, M.; Batool, F.; Iqbal, N.; Ikram ul, H. Chapter 1—Algal-Based Biopolymers. In *Algae Based Polymers, Blends, and Composites*; Zia, K.M., Zuber, M., Ali, M., Eds.; Elsevier: Amsterdam, The Netherlands, 2017; pp. 1–31. [CrossRef]
79. Nesic, A.R.; Seslija, S.I. 19—The influence of nanofillers on physical–chemical properties of polysaccharide-based film intended for food packaging. In *Food Packaging, Grumezescu, A.M., Ed.*; Academic Press: Cambridge, MA, USA, 2017; pp. 637–697. [CrossRef]
80. Qin, Y.; Jiang, J.; Zhao, L.; Zhang, J.; Wang, F. Chapter 13—Applications of Alginate as a Functional Food Ingredient. In *Biopolymers for Food Design*; Grumezescu, A.M., Holban, A.M., Eds.; Academic Press: Cambridge, MA, USA, 2018; pp. 409–429. [CrossRef]
81. Bi, D.; Li, X.; Li, T.; Li, X.; Lin, Z.; Yao, L.; Li, H.; Xu, H.; Hu, Z.; Zhang, Z.; et al. Characterization and Neuroprotection Potential of Seleno-Polymannuronate. *Front. Pharmacol.* **2020**, *11*, 21. [CrossRef]
82. El-Missiry, M.A.; Othman, A.I.; Amer, M.A.; Sedki, M.; Ali, S.M.; El-Sherbiny, I.M. Nanoformulated ellagic acid ameliorates pentylenetetrazol-induced experimental epileptic seizures by modulating oxidative stress, inflammatory cytokines and apoptosis in the brains of male mice. *Metab. Brain Dis.* **2020**, *35*, 385–399. [CrossRef]
83. Hariyadi, D.M.; Rahmadi, M.; Rahman, Z. In vivo neuroprotective activity of erythropoietin-alginate microspheres at different polymer concentrations. *Asian J. Pharm.* **2018**, *12*, 255–260.
84. Nazemi, Z.; Nourbakhsh, M.S.; Kiani, S.; Heydari, Y.; Ashtiani, M.K.; Daemi, H.; Baharvand, H. Co-delivery of minocycline and paclitaxel from injectable hydrogel for treatment of spinal cord injury. *J. Control. Release* **2020**, *321*, 145–158. [CrossRef]
85. Barrett, B. Chapter 18—Viral Upper Respiratory Infection. In *Integrative Medicine*, 4th ed.; Rakel, D., Ed.; Elsevier: Amsterdam, The Netherlands, 2018; pp. 170–179. [CrossRef]

86. Jamwal, S.; Kumar, P. Chapter 19—Animal Models of Inflammatory Bowel Disease. In *Animal Models for the Study of Human Disease*, 2nd ed.; Conn, P.M., Ed.; Academic Press: Cambridge, MA, USA, 2017; pp. 467–477. [CrossRef]
87. BeMiller, J.N. 13—Carrageenans. In *Carbohydrate Chemistry for Food Scientists (Third Edition)*, BeMiller, J.N., Ed.; AACC International Press: Eagan, MN, USA, 2019; pp. 279–291. [CrossRef]
88. Suner, S.S.; Sahiner, M.; Sengel, S.B.; Rees, D.J.; Reed, W.F.; Sahiner, N. 17—Responsive biopolymer-based microgels/nanogels for drug delivery applications. In *Stimuli Responsive Polymeric Nanocarriers for Drug Delivery Applications*; Makhlouf, A.S.H., Abu-Thabit, N.Y., Eds.; Woodhead Publishing: Sawton, Camrbide, UK, 2018; Volume 1, pp. 453–500. [CrossRef]
89. Li, R.; Wu, G. Chapter 5—Preparation of polysaccharide-based hydrogels via radiation technique. In *Hydrogels Based on Natural Polymers*; Chen, Y., Ed.; Elsevier: Amsterdam, The Netherlands, 2020; pp. 119–148. [CrossRef]
90. Wang, H.-M.D.; Li, X.-C.; Lee, D.-J.; Chang, J.-S. Potential biomedical applications of marine algae. *Bioresour. Technol.* **2017**, *244*, 1407–1415. [CrossRef]
91. Guedes, A.C.; Amaro, H.M.; Sousa-Pinto, I.; Malcata, F.X. Chapter 16—Algal spent biomass—A pool of applications. In *Biofuels from Algae*, 2nd ed.; Pandey, A., Chang, J.-S., Soccol, C.R., Lee, D.-J., Chisti, Y., Eds.; Elsevier: Amsterdam, The Netherlands, 2019; pp. 397–433. [CrossRef]
92. Zhang, H.; Zhang, F.; Yuan, R. Chapter 13—Applications of natural polymer-based hydrogels in the food industry. In *Hydrogels Based on Natural Polymers*; Chen, Y., Ed.; Elsevier: Amsterdam, The Netherlands, 2020; pp. 357–410. [CrossRef]
93. Mohanraj, R. Chapter 2—Plant-derived resorbable polymers in tissue engineering. In *Materials for Biomedical Engineering*; Grumezescu, V., Grumezescu, A.M., Eds.; Elsevier: Amsterdam, The Netherlands, 2019; pp. 19–40. [CrossRef]
94. Sudhakar, Y.N.; Selvakumar, M.; Bhat, D.K. Chapter 4—Biopolymer Electrolytes for Solar Cells and Electrochemical Cells. In *Biopolymer Electrolytes*; Sudhakar, Y.N., Selvakumar, M., Bhat, D.K., Eds.; Elsevier: Amsterdam, The Netherlands, 2018; pp. 117–149. [CrossRef]
95. Shanmugam, H.; Sathasivam, R.; Rathinam, R.; Arunkumar, K.; Carvalho, I.S. Chapter 3—Algal Biotechnology: An Update From Industrial and Medical Point of View. In *Omics Technologies and Bio-Engineering*; Barh, D., Azevedo, V., Eds.; Academic Press: Cambridge, MA, USA, 2018; pp. 31–52. [CrossRef]
96. Zoratto, N.; Matricardi, P. 4—Semi-IPNs and IPN-based hydrogels. In *Polymeric Gels*; Pal, K., Banerjee, I., Eds.; Woodhead Publishing: Sawton, Camrbide, UK, 2018; pp. 91–124. [CrossRef]
97. Qin, Y. 1—Seaweed Bioresources. In *Bioactive Seaweeds for Food Applications*; Qin, Y., Ed.; Academic Press: Cambridge, MA, USA, 2018; pp. 3–24. [CrossRef]
98. Blakemore, W.R. Polysaccharide Ingredients: Carrageenan. In *Reference Module in Food Science*; Elsevier: Amsterdam, The Netherlands, 2016. [CrossRef]
99. Qin, Y. 3—Production of Seaweed-Derived Food Hydrocolloids. In *Bioactive Seaweeds for Food Applications*; Qin, Y., Ed.; Academic Press: Cambridge, MA, USA, 2018; pp. 53–69. [CrossRef]
100. Souza, R.B.; Frota, A.F.; Silva, J.; Alves, C.; Neugebauer, A.Z.; Pinteus, S.; Rodrigues, J.A.G.; Cordeiro, E.M.S.; de Almeida, R.R.; Pedrosa, R.; et al. In vitro activities of kappa-carrageenan isolated from red marine alga Hypnea musciformis: Antimicrobial, anticancer and neuroprotective potential. *Int. J. Biol. Macromol.* **2018**, *112*, 1248–1256. [CrossRef] [PubMed]
101. Wang, Y.; Xing, M.; Cao, Q.; Ji, A.; Liang, H.; Song, S. Biological Activities of Fucoidan and the Factors Mediating Its Therapeutic Effects: A Review of Recent Studies. *Mar. Drugs* **2019**, *17*, 183. [CrossRef] [PubMed]
102. Sang, V.T.; Ngo, D.-H.; Kang, K.H.; Jung, W.-K.; Kim, S.J. The beneficial properties of marine polysaccharides in alleviation of allergic responses. *Mol. Nutr. Food Res.* **2015**, *59*, 129–138.
103. Gokarneshan, N. 19—Application of natural polymers and herbal extracts in wound management. In *Advanced Textiles for Wound Care*, 2nd ed.; Rajendran, S., Ed.; Woodhead Publishing: Sawton, Cambridge, UK, 2019; pp. 541–561. [CrossRef]
104. Gao, Y.; Zhang, L.; Jiao, W. Chapter Seven—Marine glycan-derived therapeutics in China. In *Progress in Molecular Biology and Translational Science*; Zhang, L., Ed.; Academic Press: Cambridge, MA, USA, 2019; Volume 163, pp. 113–134.

105. Wang, J.; Geng, L.; Yue, Y.; Zhang, Q. Chapter Six—Use of fucoidan to treat renal diseases: A review of 15 years of clinic studies. In *Progress in Molecular Biology and Translational Science*; Zhang, L., Ed.; Academic Press: Cambridge, MA, USA, 2019; Volume 163, pp. 95–111.
106. Park, S.K.; Kang, J.Y.; Kim, J.M.; Park, S.H.; Kwon, B.S.; Kim, G.H.; Heo, H.J. Protective effect of fucoidan extract from Ecklonia cava on hydrogen peroxide-induced neurotoxicity. *J. Microbiol. Biotechnol.* **2018**, *28*, 40–49. [CrossRef] [PubMed]
107. Hsieh, C.H.; Lu, C.H.; Kuo, Y.Y.; Lin, G.B.; Chao, C.Y. The protective effect of non-invasive low intensity pulsed electric field and fucoidan in preventing oxidative stress-induced motor neuron death via ROCK/Akt pathway. *PLoS ONE* **2019**, *14*, e0214100. [CrossRef]
108. Huang, C.Y.; Kuo, C.H.; Chen, P.W. Compressional-puffing pretreatment enhances neuroprotective effects of fucoidans from the brown seaweed sargassum hemiphyllum on 6-hydroxydopamine-induced apoptosis in SH-SY5Y cells. *Molecules* **2018**, *23*, 78. [CrossRef]
109. Alghazwi, M.; Smid, S.; Karpiniec, S.; Zhang, W. Comparative study on neuroprotective activities of fucoidans from Fucus vesiculosus and Undaria pinnatifida. *Int. J. Biol. Macromol.* **2019**, *122*, 255–264. [CrossRef]
110. Zhang, L.; Hao, J.; Zheng, Y.; Su, R.; Liao, Y.; Gong, X.; Liu, L.; Wang, X. Fucoidan protects dopaminergic neurons by enhancing the mitochondrial function in a rotenone-induced rat model of parkinson's disease. *Aging Dis.* **2018**, *9*, 590–604. [CrossRef]
111. Ahn, J.H.; Shin, M.C.; Kim, D.W.; Kim, H.; Song, M.; Lee, T.K.; Lee, J.C.; Kim, H.; Cho, J.H.; Kim, Y.M.; et al. Antioxidant properties of fucoidan alleviate acceleration and exacerbation of hippocampal neuronal death following transient global cerebral ischemia in high-fat diet-induced obese gerbils. *Int. J. Mol. Sci.* **2019**, *20*, 554. [CrossRef]
112. Kim, H.; Ahn, J.H.; Song, M.; Kim, D.W.; Lee, T.K.; Lee, J.C.; Kim, Y.M.; Kim, J.D.; Cho, J.H.; Hwang, I.K.; et al. Pretreated fucoidan confers neuroprotection against transient global cerebral ischemic injury in the gerbil hippocampal CA1 area via reducing of glial cell activation and oxidative stress. *Biomed. Pharmacother.* **2019**, *109*, 1718–1727. [CrossRef]
113. Lee, T.K.; Ahn, J.H.; Park, C.W.; Kim, B.; Park, Y.E.; Lee, J.C.; Park, J.H.; Yang, G.E.; Shin, M.C.; Cho, J.H.; et al. Pre-treatment with laminarin protects hippocampal CA1 pyramidal neurons and attenuates reactive gliosis following transient forebrain ischemia in gerbils. *Mar. Drugs* **2020**, *18*. [CrossRef] [PubMed]
114. Kumari, A. Chapter 15—Mucopolysaccharidoses. In *Sweet Biochemistry*; Kumari, A., Ed.; Academic Press: Cambridge, MA, USA, 2018; pp. 75–84. [CrossRef]
115. Duan, J.; Amster, I.J. Chapter 20—Application of FTMS to the analysis of glycosaminoglycans. In *Fundamentals and Applications of Fourier Transform Mass Spectrometry*; Kanawati, B., Schmitt-Kopplin, P., Eds.; Elsevier: Amsterdam, The Netherlands, 2019; pp. 623–649. [CrossRef]
116. Tripathy, N.; Ahmad, R.; Song, J.E.; Khang, G. Biomimetic Approaches for Regenerative Engineering. In *Encyclopedia of Biomedical Engineering*; Narayan, R., Ed.; Elsevier: Amsterdam, The Netherlands, 2019; pp. 483–495. [CrossRef]
117. Letourneau, P.C. Axonal Pathfinding: Extracellular Matrix Role. In *Reference Module in Neuroscience and Biobehavioral Psychology*; Elsevier: Amsterdam, The Netherlands, 2017. [CrossRef]
118. Vázquez, J.A.; Fraguas, J.; Novoa-Carvallal, R.; Reis, R.L.; Antelo, L.T.; Pérez-Martín, R.I.; Valcarcel, J. Isolation and chemical characterization of chondroitin sulfate from cartilage by-products of blackmouth catshark (Galeus melastomus). *Mar. Drugs* **2018**, *16*, 344. [CrossRef] [PubMed]
119. Heinegård, D.; Lorenzo, P.; Önnerfjord, P.; Saxne, T. 5—Articular cartilage. In *Rheumatology*, 6th ed.; Hochberg, M.C., Silman, A.J., Smolen, J.S., Weinblatt, M.E., Weisman, M.H., Eds.; Elsevier: Philadelphia, PA, USA, 2015; pp. 33–41. [CrossRef]
120. Chircov, C.; Grumezescu, A.M.; Bejenaru, L.E. Hyaluronic acid-based scaffolds for tissue engineering. *Rom. J. Morphol. Embryol.* **2018**, *59*, 71–76.
121. Silva, A.L.; Moura, L.I.F.; Carreira, B.; Conniot, J.; Matos, A.I.; Peres, C.; Sainz, V.; Silva, L.C.; Gaspar, R.S.; Florindo, H.F. Chapter 14—Functional Moieties for Intracellular Traffic of Nanomaterials. In *Biomedical Applications of Functionalized Nanomaterials*; Sarmento, B., das Neves, J., Eds.; Elsevier: Amsterdam, The Netherlands, 2018; pp. 399–448. [CrossRef]
122. Frisbie, D.D. 13—Hyaluronan. In *Joint Disease in the Horse*, 2nd ed.; McIlwraith, C.W., Frisbie, D.D., Kawcak, C.E., van Weeren, P.R., Eds.; W.B. Saunders: Edinburgh, Scotland, 2016; pp. 215–219. [CrossRef]

123. Kumar, S.; Ali, J.; Baboota, S. 16—Polysaccharide nanoconjugates for drug solubilization and targeted delivery. In *Polysaccharide Carriers for Drug Delivery*; Maiti, S., Jana, S., Eds.; Woodhead Publishing: Sawton, Cambridge, UK, 2019; pp. 443–475. [CrossRef]
124. Hu, M.-Y.; Nukavarapu, S. 11—Scaffolds for cartilage tissue engineering. In *Handbook of Tissue Engineering Scaffolds: Volume One*; Mozafari, M., Sefat, F., Atala, A., Eds.; Woodhead Publishing: Sawton, Cambridge, UK, 2019; pp. 211–244. [CrossRef]
125. Giji, S.; Arumugam, M. Chapter Four—Isolation and Characterization of Hyaluronic Acid from Marine Organisms. In *Advances in Food and Nutrition Research*; Kim, S.-K., Ed.; Academic Press: Cambridge, MA, USA, 2014; Volume 72, pp. 61–77.
126. Abdallah, M. Extraction of hyaluronic acid and chondroitin sulfate from marine biomass for their application in the treatment of the dry eye disease. *Acta Ophthalmol.* **2019**, *97*. [CrossRef]
127. Ho, M.T.; Teal, C.J.; Shoichet, M.S. A hyaluronan/methylcellulose-based hydrogel for local cell and biomolecule delivery to the central nervous system. *Brain Res. Bull.* **2019**, *148*, 46–54. [CrossRef]
128. He, Z.; Zang, H.; Zhu, L.; Huang, K.; Yi, T.; Zhang, S.; Cheng, S. An anti-inflammatory peptide and brain-derived neurotrophic factor-modified hyaluronan-methylcellulose hydrogel promotes nerve regeneration in rats with spinal cord injury. *Int. J. Nanomed.* **2019**, *14*, 721–732. [CrossRef]
129. Blanco, S.; Peralta, S.; Morales, M.E.; Martínez-Lara, E.; Pedrajas, J.R.; Castán, H.; Peinado, M.Á.; Ruiz, M.A. Hyaluronate nanoparticles as a delivery system to carry neuroglobin to the brain after stroke. *Pharmaceutics* **2020**, *12*. [CrossRef]
130. Nurunnabi, M.; Revuri, V.; Huh, K.M.; Lee, Y.-k. Chapter 14—Polysaccharide based nano/microformulation: An effective and versatile oral drug delivery system. In *Nanostructures for Oral Medicine*; Andronescu, E., Grumezescu, A.M., Eds.; Elsevier: Amsterdam, The Netherlands, 2017; pp. 409–433. [CrossRef]
131. Rimondo, S.; Perale, G.; Rossi, F. 6—Polysaccharide-based scaffold for tissue-regeneration. In *Functional Polysaccharides for Biomedical Applications*; Maiti, S., Jana, S., Eds.; Woodhead Publishing: Sawton, Cambridge, UK, 2019; pp. 189–212. [CrossRef]
132. Lee, S. Chapter 4—Strategic Design of Delivery Systems for Nutraceuticals. In *Nanotechnology Applications in Food*; Oprea, A.E., Grumezescu, A.M., Eds.; Academic Press: Cambridge, MA, USA, 2017; pp. 65–86. [CrossRef]
133. Vázquez, J.A.; Rodríguez-Amado, I.; Montemayor, M.I.; Fraguas, J.; González, M.D.P.; Murado, M.A. Chondroitin Sulfate, Hyaluronic Acid and Chitin/Chitosan Production Using Marine Waste Sources: Characteristics, Applications and Eco-Friendly Processes: A Review. *Mar. Drugs* **2013**, *11*, 747–774. [CrossRef]
134. Khwaldia, K. Chapter 2.3—Chondroitin and Glucosamine. In *Nonvitamin and Nonmineral Nutritional Supplements*; Nabavi, S.M., Silva, A.S., Eds.; Academic Press: Cambridge, MA, USA, 2019; pp. 27–35. [CrossRef]
135. Bougatef, H.; Krichen, F.; Capitani, F.; Amor, I.B.; Maccari, F.; Mantovani, V.; Galeotti, F.; Volpi, N.; Bougatef, A.; Sila, A. Chondroitin sulfate/dermatan sulfate from corb (*Sciaena umbra*) skin: Purification, structural analysis and anticoagulant effect. *Carbohydr. Polym.* **2018**, *196*, 272–278. [CrossRef]
136. Konovalova, I.; Novikov, V.; Kuchina, Y.; Dolgopiatova, N. Technology and Properties of Chondroitin Sulfate from Marine Hydrobionts. *KnE Life Sciences* **2020**. [CrossRef]
137. Gromova, O.A.; Torshin, I.Y.; Semenov, V.A.; Stakhovskaya, L.I.; Rudakov, K.V. On the neurological roles of chondroitin sulfate and glucosamine sulfate: A systematic analysis. *Nevrol. Neiropsikhiatriya Psikhosomatika* **2019**, *11*, 137–143. [CrossRef]
138. Iannuzzi, C.; Borriello, M.; D'Agostino, A.; Cimini, D.; Schiraldi, C.; Sirangelo, I. Protective effect of extractive and biotechnological chondroitin in insulin amyloid and advanced glycation end product-induced toxicity. *J. Cell. Physiol.* **2019**, *234*, 3814–3828. [CrossRef] [PubMed]
139. Zhang, Q.; Na, Z.; Cheng, Y.; Wang, F. Low-molecular-weight chondroitin sulfate attenuated injury by inhibiting oxidative stress in amyloid β-treated SH-SY5Y cells. *NeuroReport* **2018**, *29*, 1174–1179. [CrossRef] [PubMed]
140. Gao, F.; Zhao, J.; Liu, P.; Ji, D.; Zhang, L.; Zhang, M.; Li, Y.; Xiao, Y. Preparation and in vitro evaluation of multi-target-directed selenium-chondroitin sulfate nanoparticles in protecting against the Alzheimer's disease. *Int. J. Biol. Macromol.* **2020**, *142*, 265–276. [CrossRef]

141. Olgierd, B.; Sklarek, A.; Siwek, P.; Waluga, E. Chapter 11—Methods of Biomaterial-Aided Cell or Drug Delivery: Extracellular Matrix Proteins as Biomaterials. In *Stem Cells and Biomaterials for Regenerative Medicine*; Łos, M.J., Hudecki, A., Wiecheć, E., Eds.; Academic Press: Cambridge, MA, USA, 2019; pp. 163–189. [CrossRef]
142. Xu, K.; Jin, L. The role of heparin/heparan sulphate in the IFN-γ-led Arena. *Biochimie* **2020**, *170*, 1–9. [CrossRef]
143. Sekiguchi, R.; Yamada, K.M. Chapter Four—Basement Membranes in Development and Disease. In *Current Topics in Developmental Biology*; Litscher, E.S., Wassarman, P.M., Eds.; Academic Press: Cambridge, MA, USA, 2018; Volume 130, pp. 143–191.
144. Rudd, T.; Skidmore, M.A.; Yates, E.A. Chapter 12—Surface-Based Studies of Heparin/Heparan Sulfate-Protein Interactions: Considerations for Surface Immobilisation of HS/Heparin Saccharides and Monitoring Their Interactions with Binding Proteins. In *Chemistry and Biology of Heparin and Heparan Sulfate*; Garg, H.G., Linhardt, R.J., Hales, C.A., Eds.; Elsevier Science: Amsterdam, The Netherlands, 2005; pp. 345–366. [CrossRef]
145. De Pasquale, V.; Pavone, L.M. Heparan sulfate proteoglycans: The sweet side of development turns sour in mucopolysaccharidoses. *Biochim. Biophys. Acta (BBA)—Mol. Basis Dis.* **2019**, *1865*, 165539. [CrossRef]
146. Saravanan, R. Chapter Three—Isolation of Low-Molecular-Weight Heparin/Heparan Sulfate from Marine Sources. In *Advances in Food and Nutrition Research*; Kim, S.-K., Ed.; Academic Press: Cambridge, MA, USA, 2014; Volume 72, pp. 45–60.
147. Valcarcel, J.; Novoa-Carballal, R.; Pérez-Martín, R.I.; Reis, R.L.; Vázquez, J.A. Glycosaminoglycans from marine sources as therapeutic agents. *Biotechnol. Adv.* **2017**, *35*, 711–725. [CrossRef]
148. Aldairi, A.F.; Ogundipe, O.D.; Pye, D.A. Antiproliferative Activity of Glycosaminoglycan-Like Polysaccharides Derived from Marine Molluscs. *Mar. Drugs* **2018**, *16*, 63. [CrossRef]
149. Bejoy, J.; Song, L.; Wang, Z.; Sang, Q.X.; Zhou, Y.; Li, Y. Neuroprotective Activities of Heparin, Heparinase III, and Hyaluronic Acid on the Aβ42-Treated Forebrain Spheroids Derived from Human Stem Cells. *ACS Biomater. Sci. Eng.* **2018**, *4*, 2922–2933. [CrossRef]
150. Ye, Q.; Hai, K.; Liu, W.; Wang, Y.; Zhou, X.; Ye, Z.; Liu, X. Investigation of the protective effect of heparin pre-treatment on cerebral ischaemia in gerbils. *Pharm. Biol.* **2019**, *57*, 519–528. [CrossRef]
151. Khelif, Y.; Toutain, J.; Quittet, M.S.; Chantepie, S.; Laffray, X.; Valable, S.; Divoux, D.; Sineriz, F.; Pascolo-Rebouillat, E.; Papy-Garcia, D.; et al. A heparan sulfate-based matrix therapy reduces brain damage and enhances functional recovery following stroke. *Theranostics* **2018**, *8*, 5814–5827. [CrossRef]
152. Stillwell, W. Chapter 9—Basic Membrane Properties of the Fluid Mosaic Model. In *An Introduction to Biological Membranes*, 2nd ed.; Stillwell, W., Ed.; Elsevier: Amsterdam, The Netherlands, 2016; pp. 135–180. [CrossRef]
153. Marutescu, L.; Popa, M.; Saviuc, C.; Lazar, V.; Chifiriuc, M.C. 8—Botanical pesticides with virucidal, bactericidal, and fungicidal activity. In *New Pesticides and Soil Sensors*; Grumezescu, A.M., Ed.; Academic Press: Cambridge, MA, USA, 2017; pp. 311–335. [CrossRef]
154. Kalač, P. Chapter 4—Health-Stimulating Compounds and Effects. In *Edible Mushrooms*; Kalač, P., Ed.; Academic Press: Cambridge, MA, USA, 2016; pp. 137–153. [CrossRef]
155. Castro, R.; Tafalla, C. 2—Overview of fish immunity. In *Mucosal Health in Aquaculture*; Beck, B.H., Peatman, E., Eds.; Academic Press: Cambridge, MA, USA, 2015; pp. 3–54. [CrossRef]
156. Samoilova, N.A.; Krayukhina, M.A.; Popov, D.A.; Anuchina, N.M.; Piskarev, V.E. 3'-sialyllactose-decorated silver nanoparticles: Lectin binding and bactericidal properties. *Biointerface Res. Appl. Chem.* **2018**, *8*, 3095–3099.
157. Randy, C.; Wong, J.; Pan, W.; Chan, Y.; Yin, C.; Dan, X.; Ng, T. Marine lectins and their medicinal applications. *Appl. Microbiol. Biotechnol.* **2015**, *99*, 3755–3773.
158. Marques, D.N.; Almeida, A.S.d.; Sousa, A.R.d.O.; Pereira, R.; Andrade, A.L.; Chaves, R.P.; Carneiro, R.F.; Vasconcelos, M.A.d.; Nascimento-Neto, L.G.d.; Pinheiro, U.; et al. Antibacterial activity of a new lectin isolated from the marine sponge Chondrilla caribensis. *Int. J. Biol. Macromol.* **2018**, *109*, 1292–1301. [CrossRef] [PubMed]
159. Araújo, J.R.C.; Coelho, C.B.; Campos, A.R.; de Azevedo Moreira, R.; de Oliveira Monteiro-Moreira, A.C. Animal Galectins and Plant Lectins as Tools for Studies in Neurosciences. *Curr. Neuropharmacol.* **2020**, *18*, 202–215. [CrossRef]

160. Rahimian, R.; Lively, S.; Abdelhamid, E.; Lalancette-Hebert, M.; Schlichter, L.; Sato, S.; Kriz, J. Delayed Galectin-3-Mediated Reprogramming of Microglia After Stroke is Protective. *Mol. Neurobiol.* **2019**, *56*, 6371–6385. [CrossRef]
161. Rajkovic, I.; Wong, R.; Lemarchand, E.; Rivers-Auty, J.; Rajkovic, O.; Garlanda, C.; Allan, S.M.; Pinteaux, E. Pentraxin 3 promotes long-term cerebral blood flow recovery, angiogenesis, and neuronal survival after stroke. *J. Mol. Med.* **2018**, *96*, 1319–1332. [CrossRef]
162. Lange, K.W. Omega-3 fatty acids and mental health. *Glob. Health J.* **2020**. [CrossRef]
163. McNamara, R.K.; Asch, R.H.; Lindquist, D.M.; Krikorian, R. Role of polyunsaturated fatty acids in human brain structure and function across the lifespan: An update on neuroimaging findings. *Prostaglandins Leukot. Essent. Fat. Acids* **2018**, *136*, 23–34. [CrossRef]
164. Spector, A.A.; Kim, H.-Y. Emergence of omega-3 fatty acids in biomedical research. *Prostaglandins Leukot. Essent. Fat. Acids* **2019**, *140*, 47–50. [CrossRef]
165. Ouyang, W.-C.; Sun, G.-C.; Hsu, M.-C. Omega-3 fatty acids in cause, prevention and management of violence in schizophrenia: Conceptualization and application. *Aggress. Violent Behav.* **2020**, *50*, 101347. [CrossRef]
166. Harrington, J.W.; Bora, S. Chapter 8—Autism Spectrum Disorder. In *Integrative Medicine*, 4th ed.; Rakel, D., Ed.; Elsevier: Amsterdam, The Netherlands, 2018; pp. 64–73. [CrossRef]
167. Zhang, W.; Chen, R.; Yang, T.; Xu, N.; Chen, J.; Gao, Y.; Stetler, R.A. Fatty acid transporting proteins: Roles in brain development, aging, and stroke. *Prostaglandins Leukot. Essent. Fat. Acids* **2018**, *136*, 35–45. [CrossRef] [PubMed]
168. Gupta, C.; Prakash, D. Nutraceuticals from Microbes of Marine Sources. In *Nutraceuticals-Past, Present and Future*; IntechOpen: London, UK, 2019. [CrossRef]
169. Loftsson, T.; Ilievska, B.; Asgrimsdottir, G.M.; Ormarsson, O.T.; Stefansson, E. Fatty acids from marine lipids: Biological activity, formulation and stability. *J. Drug Deliv. Sci. Technol.* **2016**, *34*, 71–75. [CrossRef]
170. Ramesh Kumar, B.; Deviram, G.; Mathimani, T.; Duc, P.A.; Pugazhendhi, A. Microalgae as rich source of polyunsaturated fatty acids. *Biocatal. Agric. Biotechnol.* **2019**, *17*, 583–588. [CrossRef]
171. El Shatshat, A.; Pham, A.T.; Rao, P.P.N. Interactions of polyunsaturated fatty acids with amyloid peptides Aβ40 and Aβ42. *Arch. Biochem. Biophys.* **2019**, *663*, 34–43. [CrossRef] [PubMed]
172. Mallick, R.; Basak, S.; Duttaroy, A.K. Docosahexaenoic acid,22:6n-3: Its roles in the structure and function of the brain. *Int. J. Dev. Neurosci.* **2019**, *79*, 21–31. [CrossRef]
173. Zhou, M.-M.; Ding, L.; Wen, M.; Che, H.-X.; Huang, J.-Q.; Zhang, T.-T.; Xue, C.-H.; Mao, X.-Z.; Wang, Y.-M. Mechanisms of DHA-enriched phospholipids in improving cognitive deficits in aged SAMP8 mice with high-fat diet. *J. Nutr. Biochem.* **2018**, *59*, 64–75. [CrossRef]
174. Zhang, Y.-P.; Brown, R.E.; Zhang, P.-C.; Zhao, Y.-T.; Ju, X.-H.; Song, C. DHA, EPA and their combination at various ratios differently modulated Aβ25-35-induced neurotoxicity in SH-SY5Y cells. *Prostaglandins Leukot. Essent. Fat. Acids* **2018**, *136*, 85–94. [CrossRef]
175. Wang, C.-C.; Wang, D.; Zhang, T.-T.; Yanagita, T.; Xue, C.-H.; Chang, Y.-G.; Wang, Y.-M. A comparative study about EPA-PL and EPA-EE on ameliorating behavioral deficits in MPTP-induced mice with Parkinson's disease by suppressing oxidative stress and apoptosis. *J. Funct. Foods* **2018**, *50*, 8–17. [CrossRef]
176. Cheng-Sánchez, I.; Sarabia, F. Chemistry and Biology of Bioactive Glycolipids of Marine Origin. *Mar. Drugs* **2018**, *16*, 294. [CrossRef]
177. Ouellette, R.J.; Rawn, J.D. 31—Lipids and Biological Membranes. In *Organic Chemistry*, 2nd ed.; Ouellette, R.J., Rawn, J.D., Eds.; Academic Press: Cambridge, MA, USA, 2018; pp. 1001–1032. [CrossRef]
178. Aerts, J.M.F.G.; Kuo, C.-L.; Lelieveld, L.T.; Boer, D.E.C.; van der Lienden, M.J.C.; Overkleeft, H.S.; Artola, M. Glycosphingolipids and lysosomal storage disorders as illustrated by gaucher disease. *Curr. Opin. Chem. Biol.* **2019**, *53*, 204–215. [CrossRef] [PubMed]
179. Vasconcelos, A.A.; Pomin, V.H. Marine Carbohydrate-Based Compounds with Medicinal Properties. *Mar. Drugs* **2018**, *16*, 233. [CrossRef] [PubMed]
180. Li, Q.; Che, H.X.; Wang, C.C.; Zhang, L.Y.; Ding, L.; Xue, C.H.; Zhang, T.T.; Wang, Y.M. Cerebrosides from Sea Cucumber Improved Aβ 1–42 -Induced Cognitive Deficiency in a Rat Model of Alzheimer's Disease. *Mol. Nutr. Food Res.* **2019**, *63*, 1816–1823.
181. Lopez, P.H.H.; Báez, B.B. Chapter Thirteen—Gangliosides in Axon Stability and Regeneration. In *Progress in Molecular Biology and Translational Science*; Schnaar, R.L., Lopez, P.H.H., Eds.; Academic Press: Cambridge, MA, USA, 2018; Volume 156, pp. 383–412.

182. Wang, X.; Tao, S.; Cong, P.; Wang, Y.; Xu, J.; Xue, C. Neuroprotection of Strongylocentrotus nudus gangliosides against Alzheimer's disease via regulation of neurite loss and mitochondrial apoptosis. *J. Funct. Foods* **2017**, *33*, 122–133. [CrossRef]
183. Zhang, J.; Li, C.; Yu, G.; Guan, H. Total synthesis and structure-activity relationship of glycoglycerolipids from marine organisms. *Mar. drugs* **2014**, *12*, 3634–3659. [CrossRef]
184. Floris, R.; Rizzo, C.; Giudice, A.L. Biosurfactants from Marine Microorganisms. In *Metabolomics-New Insights into Biology and Medicine*; IntechOpen: London, UK, 2018. [CrossRef]
185. Sun, X.-M.; Ren, L.-J.; Zhao, Q.-Y.; Ji, X.-J.; Huang, H. Microalgae for the production of lipid and carotenoids: A review with focus on stress regulation and adaptation. *Biotechnol. Biofuels* **2018**, *11*, 272. [CrossRef]
186. Sajjadi, B.; Chen, W.-Y.; Raman, A.A.A.; Ibrahim, S. Microalgae lipid and biomass for biofuel production: A comprehensive review on lipid enhancement strategies and their effects on fatty acid composition. *Renew. Sustain. Energy Rev.* **2018**, *97*, 200–232. [CrossRef]
187. Ramesh, C.; Vinithkumar, N.V.; Kirubagaran, R.; Venil, C.K.; Dufossé, L. Multifaceted applications of microbial pigments: Current knowledge, challenges and future directions for public health implications. *Microorganisms* **2019**, *7*, 186. [CrossRef]
188. Ramesh, C.; Vinithkumar, N.; Kirubagaran, R. Marine pigmented bacteria: A prospective source of antibacterial compounds. *J. Nat. Sci. Biol. Med.* **2019**, *10*, 104–113. [CrossRef]
189. Darwesh, O.M.; Barakat, K.M.; Mattar, M.Z.; Sabae, S.Z.; Hassan, S.H. Production of antimicrobial blue green pigment pyocyanin by marine Pseudomonas aeruginosa. *Biointerface Res. Appl. Chem.* **2019**, *9*, 4334–4339.
190. Pathak, J.; Mondal, S.; Ahmed, H.; Rajneesh; Singh, S.P.; Sinha, R.P. In silico study on interaction between human polo-like kinase 1 and cyanobacterial sheath pigment scytonemin by molecular docking approach. *Biointerface Res. Appl. Chem* **2019**, *9*, 4374–4378.
191. Varmira, K.; Habibi, A.; Moradi, S.; Bahramian, E. Experimental Evaluation of Airlift Photobioreactor for Carotenoid Pigments Production by Rhodotorula rubra. *Rom. Biotechnol. Lett.* **2018**, *23*, 13843–13852.
192. Torregrosa-Crespo, J.; Montero, Z.; Fuentes, J.L.; Reig García-Galbis, M.; Garbayo, I.; Vílchez, C.; Martínez-Espinosa, R.M. Exploring the Valuable Carotenoids for the Large-Scale Production by Marine Microorganisms. *Mar. Drugs* **2018**, *16*, 203. [CrossRef] [PubMed]
193. Galasso, C.; Corinaldesi, C.; Sansone, C. Carotenoids from Marine Organisms: Biological Functions and Industrial Applications. *Antioxidants* **2017**, *6*, 96. [CrossRef] [PubMed]
194. Sathasivam, R.; Ki, J.-S. A Review of the Biological Activities of Microalgal Carotenoids and Their Potential Use in Healthcare and Cosmetic Industries. *Mar. Drugs* **2018**, *16*, 26. [CrossRef] [PubMed]
195. Huang, C.; Wen, C.; Yang, M.; Gan, D.; Fan, C.; Li, A.; Li, Q.; Zhao, J.; Zhu, L.; Lu, D. Lycopene protects against t-BHP-induced neuronal oxidative damage and apoptosis via activation of the PI3K/Akt pathway. *Mol. Biol. Rep.* **2019**, *46*, 3387–3397. [CrossRef] [PubMed]
196. Liu, C.B.; Wang, R.; Yi, Y.F.; Gao, Z.; Chen, Y.Z. Lycopene mitigates β-amyloid induced inflammatory response and inhibits NF-κB signaling at the choroid plexus in early stages of Alzheimer's disease rats. *J. Nutr. Biochem.* **2018**, *53*, 66–71. [CrossRef]
197. Cao, Z.; Wang, P.; Gao, X.; Shao, B.; Zhao, S.; Li, Y. Lycopene attenuates aluminum-induced hippocampal lesions by inhibiting oxidative stress-mediated inflammation and apoptosis in the rat. *J. Inorg. Biochem.* **2019**, *193*, 143–151. [CrossRef]
198. Man, H.B.; Bi, W.P. Protective effect of lycopene in a mouse model of Parkinson's disease via reducing oxidative stress and apoptosis. *Anal. Quant. Cytopathol. Histopathol.* **2018**, *40*, 253–258.
199. Hua, Y.; Xu, N.; Ma, T.; Liu, Y.; Xu, H.; Lu, Y. Anti-inflammatory effect of lycopene on experimental spinal cord ischemia injury via cyclooxygenase-2 suppression. *NeuroImmunoModulation* **2019**, *26*, 84–92. [CrossRef]
200. Wen, S.X.; Yang, W.C.; Shen, Z.Y.; Wang, W.; Hu, M.Y. Protective effects of lycopene on cerebral vessels and neurons of hyperlipidemic model rats. *Chin. J. Pharmacol. Toxicol.* **2019**, *33*, 93–101.
201. Han, J.H.; Lee, Y.S.; Im, J.H.; Ham, Y.W.; Lee, H.P.; Han, S.B.; Hong, J.T. Astaxanthin Ameliorates Lipopolysaccharide-Induced Neuroinflammation, Oxidative Stress and Memory Dysfunction through Inactivation of the Signal Transducer and Activator of Transcription 3 Pathway. *Mar. Drugs* **2019**, *17*, 123. [CrossRef] [PubMed]
202. Rahman, S.O.; Panda, B.P.; Parvez, S.; Kaundal, M.; Hussain, S.; Akhtar, M.; Najmi, A.K. Neuroprotective role of astaxanthin in hippocampal insulin resistance induced by Aβ peptides in animal model of Alzheimer's disease. *Biomed. Pharmacother.* **2019**, *110*, 47–58. [CrossRef] [PubMed]

203. Lu, Y.; Wang, X.; Feng, J.; Xie, T.; Si, P.; Wang, W. Neuroprotective effect of astaxanthin on newborn rats exposed to prenatal maternal seizures. *Brain Res. Bull.* **2019**, *148*, 63–69. [CrossRef]
204. Alghazwi, M.; Smid, S.; Musgrave, I.; Zhang, W. In vitro studies of the neuroprotective activities of astaxanthin and fucoxanthin against amyloid beta (Aβ 1-42) toxicity and aggregation. *Neurochem. Int.* **2019**, *124*, 215–224. [CrossRef] [PubMed]
205. Rao, S.V.; Hemalatha, P.; Yetish, S.; Muralidhara, M.; Rajini, P.S. Prophylactic neuroprotective propensity of Crocin, a carotenoid against rotenone induced neurotoxicity in mice: Behavioural and biochemical evidence. *Metab. Brain Dis.* **2019**, *34*, 1341–1353. [CrossRef]
206. Haeri, P.; Mohammadipour, A.; Heidari, Z.; Ebrahimzadeh-bideskan, A. Neuroprotective effect of crocin on substantia nigra in MPTP-induced Parkinson's disease model of mice. *Anat. Sci. Int.* **2019**, *94*, 119–127. [CrossRef]
207. Wang, C.; Cai, X.; Hu, W.; Li, Z.; Kong, F.; Chen, X.; Wang, D. Investigation of the neuroprotective effects of crocin via antioxidant activities in HT22 cells and in mice with Alzheimer's disease. *Int. J. Mol. Med.* **2019**, *43*, 956–966. [CrossRef]
208. Zhou, L.; Ouyang, L.; Lin, S.; Chen, S.; Liu, Y.; Zhou, W.; Wang, X. Protective role of β-carotene against oxidative stress and neuroinflammation in a rat model of spinal cord injury. *Int. Immunopharmacol.* **2018**, *61*, 92–99. [CrossRef]

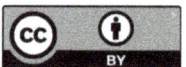

© 2020 by the authors. Licensee MDPI, Basel, Switzerland. This article is an open access article distributed under the terms and conditions of the Creative Commons Attribution (CC BY) license (http://creativecommons.org/licenses/by/4.0/).

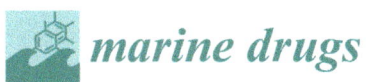

Article

Laminarin Pretreatment Provides Neuroprotection against Forebrain Ischemia/Reperfusion Injury by Reducing Oxidative Stress and Neuroinflammation in Aged Gerbils

Joon Ha Park [1,†], Ji Hyeon Ahn [2,3,†], Tae-Kyeong Lee [2], Cheol Woo Park [3], Bora Kim [3], Jae-Chul Lee [3], Dae Won Kim [4], Myoung Cheol Shin [5], Jun Hwi Cho [5], Choong-Hyun Lee [6], Soo Young Choi [2,*] and Moo-Ho Won [3,*]

1. Department of Anatomy, College of Korean Medicine, Dongguk University, Gyeongju, Gyeongbuk 38066, Korea; jh-park@dongguk.ac.kr
2. Department of Biomedical Science and Research Institute for Bioscience and Biotechnology, Hallym University, Chuncheon, Gangwon 24252, Korea; jh-ahn@hallym.ac.kr (J.H.A.); xorud312@naver.com (T.-K.L.)
3. Department of Neurobiology, School of Medicine, Kangwon National University, Chuncheon, Gangwon 24341, Korea; flfhflfh@naver.com (C.W.P.); nbrkim17@gmail.com (B.K.); anajclee@kangwon.ac.kr (J.-C.L.)
4. Department of Biochemistry and Molecular Biology, and Research Institute of Oral Sciences, College of Dentistry, Gangnung-Wonju National University, Gangneung, Gangwon 25457, Korea; kimdw@gwnu.ac.kr
5. Department of Emergency Medicine, and Institute of Medical Sciences, Kangwon National University Hospital, School of Medicine, Kangwon National University, Chuncheon, Gangwon 24341, Korea; dr10126@naver.com (M.C.S.); cjhemd@kangwon.ac.kr (J.H.C.)
6. Department of Pharmacy, College of Pharmacy, Dancook University, Cheonan, Chungcheongnam 31116, Korea; anaphy@dankook.ac.kr
* Correspondence: sychoi@hallym.ac.kr (S.Y.C.); mhwon@kangwon.ac.kr (M.-H.W.); Tel.: +82-33-248-2112 (S.Y.C.); +82-33-250-8891 (M.-H.W.); Fax: +82-33-241-1463 (S.Y.C.); +82-33-256-1614 (M.-H.W.)
† The two authors have contributed equally to this article.

Received: 17 March 2020; Accepted: 13 April 2020; Published: 15 April 2020

Abstract: Laminarin is a polysaccharide isolated from brown algae that has various biological and pharmacological activities, such as antioxidant and anti-inflammatory properties. We recently reported that pretreated laminarin exerted neuroprotection against transient forebrain ischemia/reperfusion (IR) injury when we pretreated with 50 mg/kg of laminarin once a day for seven days in adult gerbils. However, there have been no studies regarding a neuroprotective effect of pretreated laminarin against IR injury in aged animals and its related mechanisms. Therefore, in this study, we intraperitoneally inject laminarin (50 mg/kg) once a day to aged gerbils for seven days before IR (5-min transient ischemia) surgery and examine the neuroprotective effect of laminarin treatment and the mechanisms in the gerbil hippocampus. IR injury in vehicle-treated gerbils causes loss (death) of pyramidal neurons in the hippocampal CA1 field at five days post-IR. Pretreatment with laminarin effectively protects the CA1 pyramidal neurons from IR injury. Regarding the laminarin-treated gerbils, production of superoxide anions, 4-hydroxy-2-nonenal expression and pro-inflammatory cytokines [interleukin(IL)-1β and tumor necrosis factor-α] expressions are significantly decreased in the CA1 pyramidal neurons after IR. Additionally, laminarin treatment significantly increases expressions of superoxide dismutase and anti-inflammatory cytokines (IL-4 and IL-13) in the CA1 pyramidal neurons before and after IR. Taken together, these findings indicate that laminarin can protect neurons from ischemic brain injury in an aged population by attenuating IR-induced oxidative stress and neuroinflammation.

Keywords: laminarin; aging; transient cerebral ischemia; neuroprotection; oxidative stress; neuroinflammation

1. Introduction

Transient ischemia in the brain occurs when the blood supply to part of the brain or the whole brain is briefly interrupted by occlusion of regional arteries or by cardiac ischemia [1,2]. Transient brain ischemia results in irreversible and persistent damage to the brain parenchyma [3,4]. Globally, transient ischemia-induced brain injury is a major cause of death or long-term disability [5], showing that the brain injury is triggered by complex mechanisms [6,7]. Among the complex mechanisms, oxidative stress and neuroinflammation have been regarded as major contributors to the pathogenesis of ischemic brain injury following transient brain ischemia [8–10]. Therefore, inhibition of oxidative stress and neuroinflammation has been a focus of studies on developing neuroprotection against transient ischemia-induced brain injury [11,12] and neurodegenerative disease [13].

Many studies have been conducted to develop therapeutic candidates against ischemic brain injury using experimental animals; however, these studies have been carried out in adult animals [14–16]. Brain ischemia (ischemic stroke) is one of the most important age-related diseases. Approximately one third of patients with ischemic stroke are in the aged population [17]. Due to a longer life expectancy, the incidence of brain ischemia will increase further over time, and aging has been known as one of the major risk factors affecting ischemic brain injury [18–20]. Aged brains are more susceptible to ischemic brain injury, and protective efficacy against ischemic injury is low in the aged population [21]. Thus, we need to assess therapeutic strategies against ischemic brain injury in aged experimental animals.

Medicinal plant-derived natural compounds have received considerable attention as potential sources of therapeutic candidates for the prevention and treatment of neurological diseases, including brain ischemia, because they display a wide spectrum of biological properties [22,23]. Marine algae-derived compounds also have been shown to protect against brain ischemic injury. Fucoidan, for example, a type of polysaccharide extracted from various species of brown algae, shows strong neuroprotective effects against ischemic brain injury in animal models of brain ischemia [24–27]. Additionally, we recently reported that laminarin, a water-soluble polysaccharide derived from the brown algae *Laminaria digitate*, showed neuroprotection against IR brain injury in adult gerbils [28]. Laminarin exhibits biofunctional properties, such as anti-apoptotic [29], anti-oxidant [30], anti-inflammatory [31], and anti-cancer [32] activities.

However, to the best of our knowledge, there have been few studies about the neuroprotective effects of laminarin against ischemic brain injury in aged experimental animals, although there is a high incidence of brain ischemia in the aged population. Additionally, the underlying mechanisms of the neuroprotective effects of laminarin against ischemic brain injury have not been fully addressed. Thus, our objective in this study is to investigate the neuroprotective effect and mechanisms of laminarin as a potential neuroprotective agent in the hippocampus of aged gerbils following brain IR injury. The hippocampus is well known as one of the brain regions most vulnerable to transient brain ischemia [33,34]. Specifically, extensive loss of pyramidal neurons takes place in the hippocampal cornu ammonis 1 (CA1) region over several days after transient ischemia in both humans and experimental animals [3,7,35].

2. Results

2.1. Protection of Neurons from IR Injury by Laminarin

2.1.1. Neuronal Nuclear Antigen (NeuN) Immunoreactive ($^+$) Cells

During the vehicle-sham and laminarin-sham groups, NeuN immunofluorescence was easily detected in intact neurons in all hippocampal subregions (Figure 1A(a,e)), and this finding was not different from that in the control group (data not shown). Regarding the hippocampus proper [cornu ammonis 1(CA1)–CA3], pyramidal cells, which consist of the striatum pyramidal, showed strong NeuN immunofluorescence (Figure 1A(a,b,e,f)).

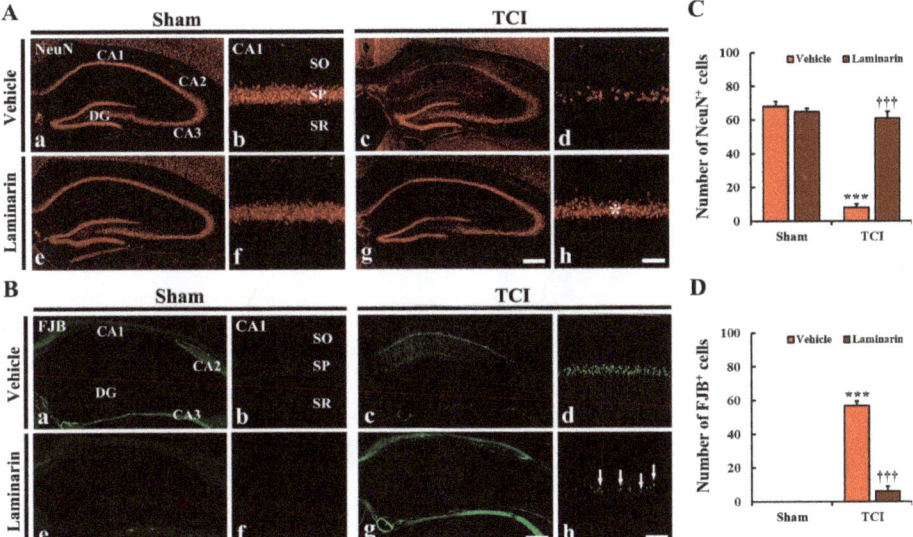

Figure 1. (**A**,**B**) Representative images of NeuN immunofluorescence (**A**) and FJB histofluorescence staining (**B**) in CA1 of the vehicle-sham (**a**,**b**), vehicle-IR (**c**,**d**), laminarin-sham (**e**,**f**), and laminarin-IR (**g**,**h**) groups at five days after IR. Regarding the vehicle-IR group, a few NeuN$^+$ and many FJB$^+$ cells are shown in the stratum pyramidal (SP). However, in the laminarin-IR group, numerous NeuN$^+$ cells (asterisk) and a few FJB$^+$ cells (arrows) are shown in the SP. CA, cornu ammonis; DG, dentate gyrus; FJB, Fluoro-Jade B; NeuN, nuclear antigen; SO, stratum oriens; SR, stratum radiatum. Scale bar = 400 µm (**a**,**c**,**e**,**g**), 50 µm (**b**,**d**,**f**,**h**). (**C**,**D**) Mean number of NeuN$^+$ (**C**) and FJB$^+$ cells (**D**) in CA1. The bars indicate means ± SEM (n = 7/group; *** $p < 0.001$ versus each sham group, $^{+++}$ $p < 0.001$ versus vehicle-IR group).

Concerning the vehicle-IR group, NeuN$^+$ pyramidal cells were significantly decreased in number in CA1, but not in CA2/3, at five days post-IR (Figure 1A(c,d)). Then, the number of NeuN$^+$ CA1 pyramidal cells was 8.4 ± 2.2 cells/200 × 200 µm (Figure 1C). However, in the laminarin-IR group, a considerable number of NeuN$^+$ CA1 pyramidal cells (61.3 ± 4.1 cells/200 × 200 µm) was observed, compared to that in the vehicle-IR group (Figure 1A(g,h),C). This finding means that pretreated laminarin protected hippocampal CA1 pyramidal neurons from 5-min IR in aged gerbils.

2.1.2. Fluoro-Jade B (FJB)$^+$ Cells

Concerning the vehicle-sham and laminarin-sham groups, FJB$^+$ cells, which are dead cells, were not detected in the hippocampus (Figure 1B(a,b,e,f)). Also, similar results were obtained in the control group of animals (data not shown).

Regarding the vehicle-IR group, numerous FJB$^+$ cells were shown in the stratum pyramidal of CA1 at five days post-IR (Figure 1B(c,d)), showing that the number of FJB$^+$ CA1 pyramidal cells was 57.6 ± 2.5 cells/200 × 200 µm (Figure 1D). Concerning the laminarin-IR group, only a few FJB$^+$ CA1 pyramidal cells (6.4 ± 3.3 cells/200 × 200 µm) were shown in CA1, compared to those in the vehicle-IR group (Figure 1B(g,h),D).

2.2. Increases of Superoxide Dismutase (SODs) Expression by Laminarin

Regarding the vehicle-sham group, copper-zinc SOD (SOD1) and manganese SOD (SOD2) immunoreactivity were easily shown in CA1 pyramidal cells (Figure 2A(a),B(a)). Concerning the vehicle-IR group, SOD1 and SOD2 immunoreactivity in the CA1 pyramidal cells were significantly decreased at one day post-IR (by about 24% and 22%, respectively) compared to that in the vehicle-sham group (Figure 2A(b),B(b),C,D), and, at five days post-IR, SOD1 and SOD2 immunoreactivity were significantly decreased further (about 25% and 34% of the vehicle-sham group, respectively) (Figure 2A(c),B(c),C,D).

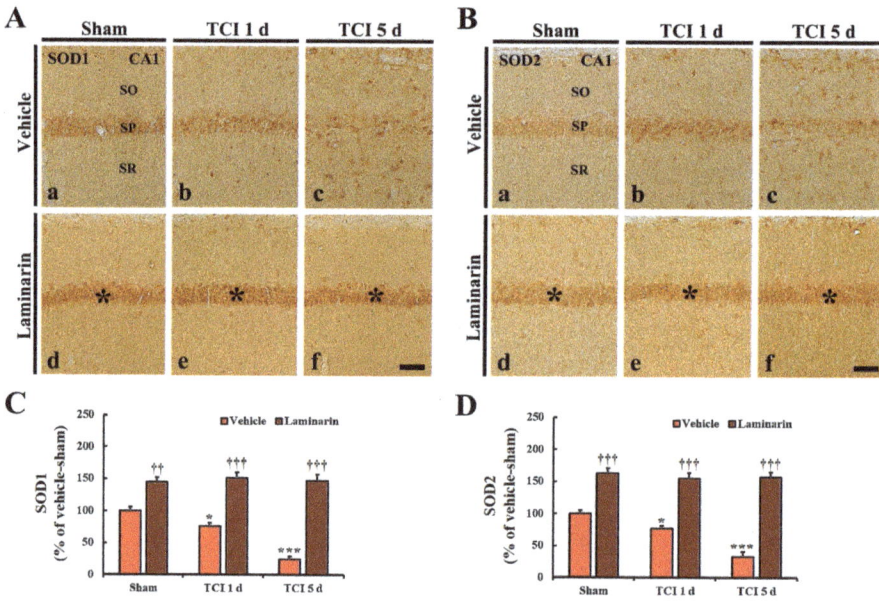

Figure 2. (**A,B**) Images of immunochemistry for SOD1 (**A**) and SOD2 (**B**) in CA1 of the vehicle-sham (**a**), vehicle-IR (**b,c**), laminarin-sham (**d**), and laminarin-IR (**e,f**) groups at one day (**b,e**) and five days (**c,f**) after IR. Regarding the vehicle-IR group, SOD1 and SOD2 immunoreactivity are significantly increased with time in the stratum pyramidale (SP). Concerning the laminarin-sham group, SOD1 and SOD2 immunoreactivity in the SP (asterisks) are significantly higher than that in the vehicle-sham group. Regarding the laminarin-IR group, both immunoreactivities (asterisks) are sustained until five days post-IR. SOD, superoxide dismutase; SO, stratum oriens; SR, stratum radiatum. Scale bar = 50 μm. (**C,D**) Relative immunoreactivity (RI) of SOD1 (**C**) and SOD2 (**D**) immunoreactivity in CA1 pyramidal cells. The bars indicate the means ± SEM ($n = 7$/group; * $p < 0.05$, *** $p < 0.001$ versus each sham group, †† $p < 0.01$, ††† $p < 0.001$ versus vehicle-IR group).

Seen in the laminarin-sham group, SOD1 and SOD2 immunoreactivity in CA1 pyramidal cells were significantly higher (about 145% and 163%, respectively) than that in the vehicle-sham group (Figure 2A(d),B(d),C,D). Interestingly, in the laminarin-IR group, the increased SOD1 and SOD2 immunoreactivity were sustained until five days post-IR (Figure 2A(e,f),B(e,f),C,D).

2.3. Attenuation of IR-Induced Oxidative Stress by Laminarin

2.3.1. Dihydroethidium (DHE) Fluorescence

Weak DHE fluorescence was detected in CA1 pyramidal cells of the vehicle-sham group (Figure 3Aa). Regarding the vehicle-IR group, DHE fluorescence intensity in the CA1 pyramidal cells was significantly increased by about 333% at one day post-IR and by about 269% at five days post-IR, compared with that in the vehicle-sham group (Figure 3A(b,c),C). Particularly, at one and five days post-IR, strong DHE fluorescence was shown in many non-pyramidal cells located in strata oriens and radiatum (Figure 3A(b,c)).

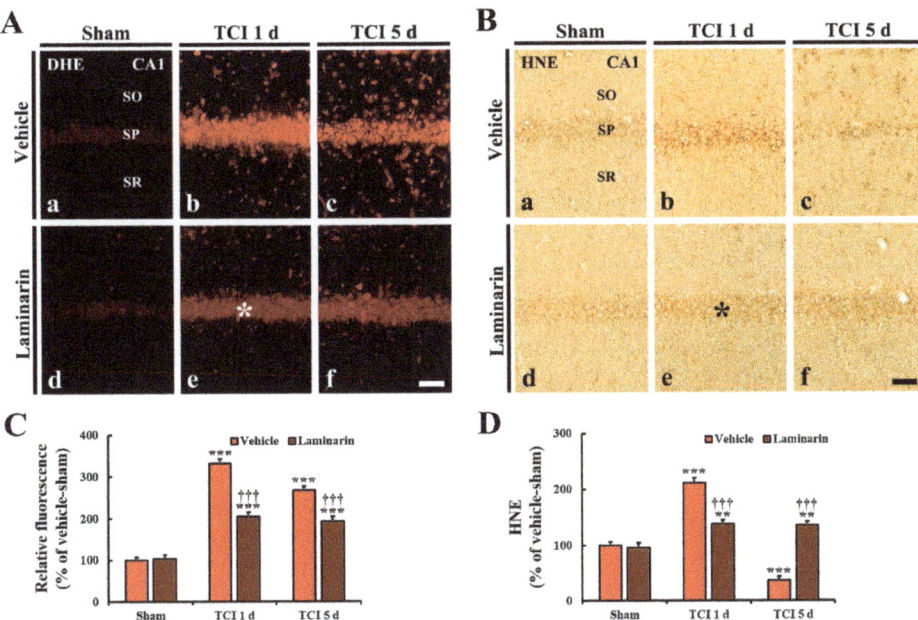

Figure 3. (**A**,**B**) DHE fluorescence staining (**A**) and HNE immunohistochemistry (**B**) in CA1 of the vehicle-sham (**a**), vehicle-IR (**b**,**c**), laminarin-sham (**d**), and laminarin-IR (**e**,**f**) groups at one day (**b**,**e**) and five days (**c**,**f**) after IR. Regarding the vehicle-IR group, DHE fluorescence and HNE immunoreactivity in the stratum pyramidale (SP) are significantly increased at one day post-IR and decreased at five days post-IR. Concerning the laminarin-IR group, DHE fluorescence (asterisk) and HNE immunoreactivity (asterisk) at one day post-IR are significantly lower than those in the vehicle-IR group, and, at five days post-IR, DHE fluorescence and HNE immunoreactivity are maintained. Dihydroethidium, DHE; 4-hydroxy-2-nonenal, HNE; SO, stratum oriens; SR, stratum radiatum. Scale bar = 50 μm. (**C**,**D**) Relative immunoreactivity (RI) of DHE fluorescence (**C**) and HNE immunoreactivity (**D**) in CA1 pyramidal cells. The bars indicate the mean ± SEM ($n = 7$/group; ** $p < 0.01$, *** $p < 0.001$ versus each sham group, ††† $p < 0.001$ versus vehicle-IR group).

Concerning the laminarin-sham group, DHE fluorescence and its intensity in CA1 pyramidal cells were not different from those in the vehicle-sham group (Figure 3A(d),C). However, in the laminarin-IR group, DHE fluorescence intensity at one day post-IR was significantly lower compared with that in the vehicle-IR group (about 62% of the vehicle-IR group), and the DHE fluorescence intensity was sustained until five days post-IR (Figure 3A(e,f),C).

2.3.2. 4-Hydroxy-2-Nonenal (HNE) Immunoreactivity

Regarding the vehicle-sham group, weak HNE immunoactivity was detected in CA1 pyramidal cells (Figure 3B(a)). Concerning the vehicle-IR group, HNE immunoreactivity in the CA1 pyramidal cells was significantly increased (by about 212%) at one day post-IR compared with that of the vehicle-sham group and, at five days post-IR, its immunoreactivity was very low because the CA1 pyramidal cells were dead by IR (Figure 3B(b,c),D).

Regarding the laminarin-sham group, HNE immunoreactivity in CA1 pyramidal cells was similar to that in the vehicle-sham group (Figure 3B(d),D). Concerning the laminarin-IR group, HNE immunoreactivity in the CA1 pyramidal cells was significantly low at one day post-IR compared with that in the vehicle-IR group (about 73% of the vehicle-IR group), and its immunoreactivity was not altered until five days post-IR (Figure 3B(e,f),D).

2.4. Reduction of IR-Induced Neuroinflammation by Laminarin

2.4.1. Pro-Inflammatory Cytokine Immunoreactivities

Interleukin (IL)-1β and tumor necrosis factor (TNF)α immunoreactivities in the vehicle-sham group were observed in CA1 pyramidal cells (Figure 4A(a),B(a)). Regarding the vehicle-IR group, IL-1β and TNFα immunoreactivities in the CA1 pyramidal cells were significantly increased (by about 186% and 195%, respectively) at one day post-IR compared with that in the vehicle-sham group (Figure 4A(b),B(b),C,D). Occurring by five days post-IR, each immunoreactivity was very low in CA1 pyramidal cells due to damage to the CA1 pyramidal cells by IR (Figure 4A(c),B(c),C,D).

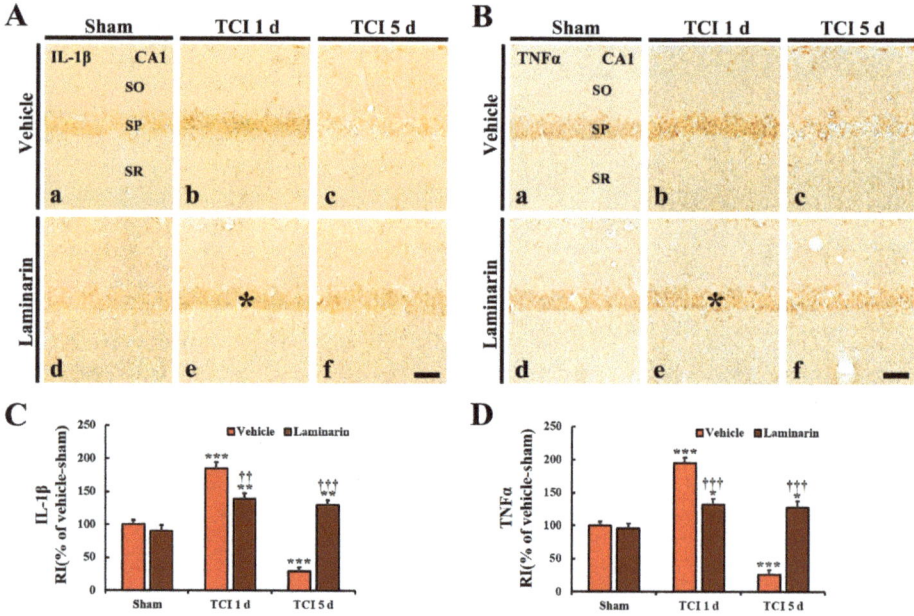

Figure 4. (**A,B**) Immunochemistry for IL-1β (**A**) and TNFα (**B**) in CA1 of the vehicle-sham (**a**), vehicle-IR (**b,c**), laminarin-sham (**d**), and laminarin-IR (**e,f**) groups at one day (**b,e**) and five days (**c,f**) after IR. Regarding the vehicle-IR group, IL-1β and TNFα immunoreactivities are significantly increased in the stratum pyramidale (SP) (asterisks) and hardly shown at five days post-IR. Concerning the laminarin-IR group, IL-1β and TNFα immunoreactivities in the SP (asterisks) are significantly lower than those in the vehicle-IR group at one day post-IR and not changed at five days post-IR. Interleukin, IL; tumor necrosis factor, TNF; SO, stratum oriens; SR, stratum radiatum. Scale bar = 50 μm. (**C,D**) Relative immunoreactivity (RI) of IL-1β (**C**) and TNFα (**D**) immunoreactivity in CA1 pyramidal cells. The bars indicate the means ± SEM ($n = 7$/group; * $p < 0.05$, ** $p < 0.01$, *** $p < 0.001$ versus each sham group, †† $p < 0.01$, ††† $p < 0.001$ versus vehicle-IR group).

Regarding the laminarin-sham group, IL-1β and TNFα immunoreactivities in CA1 pyramidal cells were similar to those in the vehicle-sham group (Figure 4A(d),B(d),C,D). However, in the laminarin-IR group, IL-1β and TNFα immunoreactivities in the CA1 pyramidal cells were significantly lower (about

43% and 73%, respectively) at one day post-IR than those in the vehicle-IR group (Figure 4A(e),B(e),C,D), and each immunoreactivity was not changed until five days post-IR (Figure 4A(f),B(f),C,D).

2.4.2. Anti-Inflammatory Cytokine Immunoreactivities

IL-4 and IL-13 immunoreactivities were found in CA1 pyramidal cells in the vehicle-sham group (Figure 5A(a),B(a)). Regarding the vehicle-IR group, both IL-4 and IL-13 immunoreactivities in the CA1 pyramidal cells were significantly reduced (about 72% and 64%, respectively) at one day post-IR compared with that in the vehicle-sham group (Figure 5A(b),B(b),C,D) and, at five days post-IR, both immunoreactivities were very low due to damage (death) to the CA1 pyramidal cells by IR (Figure 5A(c),B(c),C,D).

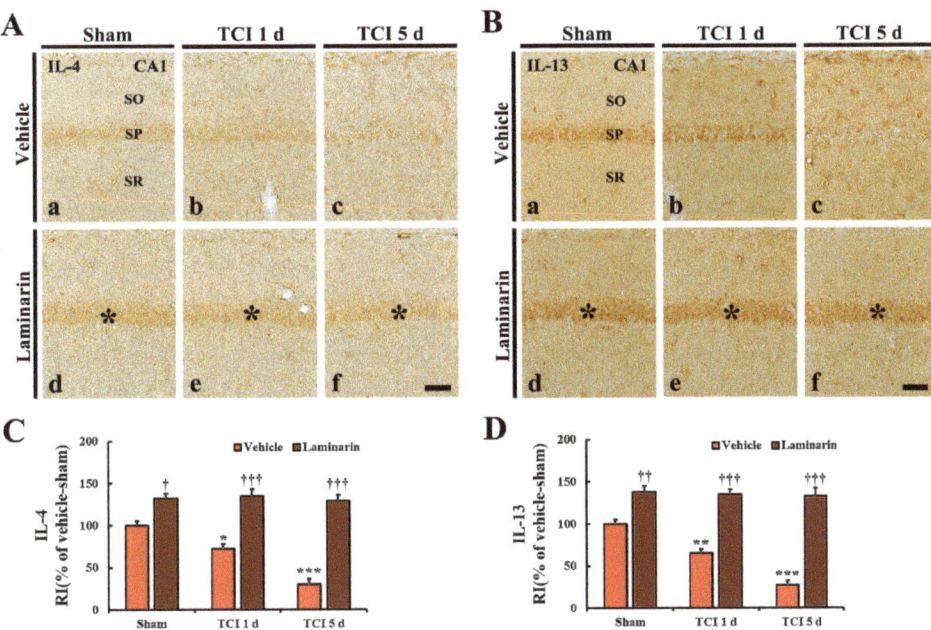

Figure 5. (**A**,**B**) Immunochemistry for IL-4 (**A**) and IL-13 (**B**) in CA1 of the vehicle-sham (**a**), vehicle-IR (**b**,**c**), laminarin-sham (**d**), and laminarin-IR (**e**,**f**) groups at one day (**b**,**e**) and five days (**c**,**f**) after IR. Regarding the vehicle-IR group, IL-4 and IL-13 immunoreactivities in the stratum pyramidale (SP) are gradually decreased after IR. Concerning the laminarin-sham group, IL-4 and IL-13 immunoreactivities in the SP (asterisks) are high compared with those in the vehicle-sham group, and the increased immunoreactivities in the SP (asterisks) are maintained until five days post-IR. IL, interleukin; SO, stratum oriens; SR, stratum radiatum. Scale bar = 50 μm. (**C**,**D**) Relative immunoreactivity (RI) of IL-4 (**C**) and IL-13 (**D**) immunoreactivity in CA1 pyramidal cells. The bars indicate the means ± SEM ($n = 7$/group; * $p < 0.05$, *** $p < 0.001$ versus each sham group, † $p < 0.05$, †† $p < 0.01$, ††† $p < 0.001$ versus vehicle-IR group).

Concerning the laminarin-sham group, IL-4, and IL-13 immunoreactivities in CA1 pyramidal cells were significantly higher (about 132% and 138%, respectively) than that in the vehicle-sham group (Figure 5A(d),B(d),C,D). Regarding the laminarin-IR group, the increased IL-4 and IL-13 immunoreactivities in the CA1 pyramidal cells were maintained at one and five days post-IR (Figure 5A(e,f),B(e,f),C,D).

3. Discussion

Pretreatment with polysaccharides isolated from brown algae elicits neuroprotective effects against ischemic brain injuries. Pretreated fucoidan, for example, significantly reduces cerebral infarction size following transient focal cerebral ischemia induced by middle cerebral artery occlusion (MCAO)in adult rats [25] and protects pyramidal neurons in the hippocampal CA1 from IR injury in an adult gerbil model of transient global forebrain ischemia [27]. Furthermore, we recently reported that laminarin pretreatment had a strong neuroprotection in the hippocampal CA1 against IR injury in an adult gerbil model of transient global forebrain ischemia [28]. However, the above-mentioned studies were done in adult animal models; these studies have a limitation in not addressing ischemic insults in the aged population with a higher risk of ischemic stroke. Thus, in this study, we evaluated how pretreatment with laminarin protects neurons in an aged gerbil hippocampus following IR by using NeuN immunofluorescence and FJB histofluorescence staining. We found that pretreatment with laminarin effectively protected CA1 pyramidal neurons from IR injury. This result indicates that laminarin could be applied as a possible candidate for prevention of ischemic stroke in the aged population.

It has been reported that the aged brain is sensitive to oxidative stress and neuroinflammation [36,37]. A growing number of studies also have suggested that oxidative stress caused by excessive production of reactive oxygen species (ROS) and neuroinflammation mediated by activation of glial cells and release of inflammatory mediators are major factors leading to neuronal death following cerebral ischemia [8,38]. Based on the above-mentioned studies, researchers have demonstrated that treatments with pharmacological agents, including natural products, alleviate ischemia-induced oxidative stress and neuroinflammation, and contribute strongly to neuroprotection against ischemic brain injury [27,39,40]. During this study, we used pretreatment of gerbils with laminarin and found that SOD1 and SOD2, as endogenous antioxidant enzymes, were markedly increased in CA1 pyramidal neurons before and after IR induction. It has been suggested that increased endogenous antioxidant enzymes prevent the accumulation of ROS [41] and can protect against ischemic injuries [42]. To investigate whether increased SODs protect neurons from IR injury, we examined levels in DHE (a probe to detect superoxide anions) and HNE (a product of lipid peroxidation), as indicators of oxidative stress in the laminarin-IR group and found they were significantly more alleviated in the CA1 pyramidal neurons than those in the vehicle-IR group. This finding means that IR-induced oxidative stress is significantly reduced by laminarin preconditioning.

Here, we found that levels of pro-inflammatory cytokines (IL-1β and TNFα) were significantly increased in the CA1 pyramidal neurons in the vehicle-IR group after IR but, in the laminarin-IR group, the increased levels of IL-1β and TNFα were significantly reduced after IR. Furthermore, anti-inflammatory cytokines (IL-4 and IL-13), which are involved in the resolution of neuroinflammation [43], were significantly increased in the CA1 pyramidal neurons in the laminarin-IR group before and after IR.

Although the protective effects of laminarin against IR-induced oxidative stress and neuroinflammation have not been addressed yet in aged brains following ischemic insults, Yao et al. (2018) recently reported that laminarin effectively delayed the aging of oocytes and improved the quality of aged oocytes by reducing the ROS level and increasing the glutathione level. Additionally, Cheng et al. (2011) reported that laminarin significantly attenuated sepsis-induced oxidative damage in the lung of the rat by reducing the malondialdehyde (MDA, an end product of lipid peroxidation) level and increasing the activities of endogenous antioxidant enzymes, such as SODs, catalase, and glutathione peroxidase. Regarding the case of inflammation, Neyrinck et al. (2007) showed that laminarin protected against LPS-induced hepatotoxicity in rats via a decrease in the serum monocyte number, nitrite, and TNFα. Additionally, we recently reported that laminarin pretreatment strongly attenuated activations of astrocytes and microglia in the hippocampal CA1 after brain IR in gerbils [28]. Thus, together with our and other previous studies, our current findings potentially suggest that alleviation of oxidative stress and neuroinflammation in the ischemic hippocampal CA1 of aged gerbils by pretreatment with laminarin contributes to neuroprotection against IR injury.

Here, we investigated IR-induced changes of oxidative stress, antioxidants (SOD1 and SOD2), and inflammatory cytokines (IL-1β, TNFα, IL-4, and IL-13) in the hippocampal CA1 region by immunohistochemistry. Regarding quantitative analyses, these factors will be examined by western blot or real-time polymerase chain reaction in the future study.

To summarize, our findings provide clear evidences that pretreatment with laminarin protects CA1 pyramidal neurons in the hippocampus from IR injury in an aged gerbil model of transient global forebrain ischemia. This effect might be closely related to attenuation of oxidative stress and neuroinflammation in the ischemic CA1 following laminarin pretreatment. Therefore, laminarin can be used as a potential candidate for attenuating ischemic brain injury in the aged population in the future, although further studies are needed to investigate much more specific molecular mechanisms.

4. Materials and Methods

4.1. Experimental Groups and Laminarin Pretreatment

Aged male gerbils (age 22–24 months [44]; body weight 80–90 g) were supplied by the Experimental Animal Center, Kangwon National University (Chuncheon, Gangwon, Korea). Animal care and handling followed the guidelines of current international laws and policies, which are in the NIH Guide for the Care and Use of Laboratory Animals (The National Academies Press, 8th Ed., 2011), and the protocol of this experiment was approved (approval number, KW- KW-200113-1) by the Institutional Animal Care and Use Committee (IACUC) of Kangwon National University.

A total of 53 gerbils were randomly assigned to five groups: (1) control group ($n = 5$); (2) vehicle-sham group ($n = 10$), which was treated with vehicle (saline) and not subjected to IR; (3) vehicle-IR group ($n = 14$), which was treated with vehicle and subjected to IR; (4) laminarin-sham group ($n = 10$), which was treated with 50 mg/kg of laminarin and not subjected to IR; (5) laminarin-IR group ($n = 14$), which was treated with 50 mg/kg of laminarin and subjected to IR. The gerbils in the experimental groups were sacrificed at 1 day and 5 days after IR surgery. The dosage and duration of laminarin (Sigma–Aldrich, Poole, Dorset, UK) treatment were selected based on the results of our previous study [28]. The vehicle and laminarin were administered intraperitoneally once a day for 7 consecutive days before IR.

4.2. Surgery of IR

Briefly, as described previously [45], the gerbils used in this study were anesthetized with a mixture of 2–3% isoflurane in 33% oxygen and 67% nitrous oxide using inhalation anesthesia equipment (Harvard Apparatus, Holliston, MA, USA). The bilateral common carotid arteries were exposed through a 2-cm ventral midline incision in their necks and simultaneously occluded for 5 min with non-traumatic aneurysm clips (Yasargil FE 723K, Aesculap, Tuttlingen, Germany). Five minutes later, the clips were removed to restore cerebral blood flow. The restoration of blood flow was directly observed through the retinal arteries, which are branches of the internal carotid arteries, with an ophthalmoscope (HEINE K180, Heine Optotechnik, Herrsching, Germany). The body temperature of each animal was checked and maintained at a normothermic condition (37 ± 0.5 °C) throughout the whole process of the experiment using a heating pad (homeothermic monitoring system, Harvard Apparatus, Holliston, MA, USA). The gerbils subjected to the sham operation received the same IR surgery without occlusion of both common carotid arteries.

4.3. Preparation of Brain Sections

As previously described [46], the animals ($n = 5$ in the control group; $n = 5$ at 1 and 5 days post-IR in each sham group; $n = 7$ at 1 and 5 days post-IT in each IR group) were intraperitoneally anesthetized with urethane (1.5 g/kg, Sigma–Aldrich, St. Louis, MO, USA) and perfused with a solution of 4%

paraformaldehyde (in 0.1 M phosphate buffer, pH 7.4). Their brains were removed and more fixed (for 6 h) with the same fixative. The fixed brains were cryoprotected by infiltration with a solution of 30% sucrose [in 0.1 M phosphate-buffered saline (PBS), pH 7.4] and coronally sectioned (30 μm thickness) in cryostat (Leica, Wetzlar, Germany).

4.4. NeuN Immunofluorescence and FJB Histofluorescence Staining

To evaluate the protection of neurons by pretreated laminarin, NeuN (a marker for neuron) immunofluorescence staining and FJB (a fluorescent marker for neuronal degeneration) histofluorescence staining were performed on the hippocampus at 5 days post-IR. Briefly, as previously described [45], the brain sections were incubated with a solution of mouse anti-NeuN (1:1000, Chemicon, Temecula, CA, USA) overnight at 4 °C. These sections were washed in PBS and reacted with a solution of Cy3-conjugated donkey anti-mouse immunoglobulin G (1:500, Vector Laboratories Inc., Burlingame, CA, USA) for 2 h at room temperature. Regarding FJB histofluorescence staining, the sections were immersed in a solution of 1% sodium hydroxide (Sigma–Aldrich, St. Louis, MO, USA), transferred to a solution of 0.06% potassium permanganate (Sigma–Aldrich, St. Louis, MO, USA) and incubated in a solution of 0.0004% FJB (Histochem, Jefferson, AR, USA). Finally, these stained sections were washed and placed on a slide warmer controlled at about 50 °C for 4 h to be reacted.

Neuroprotection was analyzed as previously described [47]. Five sections containing the hippocampus were selected with a 140-μm interval in each gerbil brain. These sections were anteroposterior from −1.4 to −2.2 mm of the gerbil brain atlas [48]. NeuN$^+$ and FJB$^+$ cells were counted as follows. Briefly, digital images of all of the cells were captured in the hippocampus with a fluorescence microscope (BX53) (Olympus, Tokyo, Japan) equipped with a digital camera (DP7) (Olympus, Tokyo, Japan) connected to a PC monitor. Both cells were captured in 200 × 200 μm^2 at the center of CA1. Each mean cell number was obtained by averaging the total numbers using an image analyzing system (Optimas 6.5) (CyberMetrics, Scottsdale, AZ, USA).

4.5. DHE Staining for Superoxide

DHE (Sigma–Aldrich, St. Louis, MO, USA) is the most popular fluorogenic probe to detect intracellular superoxide anions and is used to analyze oxidative stress. We applied DHE staining in the brain sections, as described previously [47]. Briefly, the sections were equilibrated in a Krebs–HEPES buffer (composed of 130 mM NaCl, 5.6 mM KCl, 2 mM $CaCl_2$, 0.24 mM $MgCl_2$, 8.3 mM HEPES, 11 mM glucose, pH 7.4, etc.) for 40 min at 37 °C. Fresh buffer containing DHE (10 μmol/L) was applied on the sections for 2 h at 37 °C, and DHE was oxidized upon reaction with superoxide to ethidium bromide, which binds DNA in nuclei.

Oxidative stress was analyzed based on the relative fluorescence intensity of DHE. Briefly, as described previously [27], images were captured from CA1 using a BX53 fluorescence microscope (Olympus, Tokyo, Japan) with an excitation wavelength of 520–540 nm. The DHE fluorescence intensity was analyzed using Image-pro Plus 6.0 software (Media Cybernetics, Rockville, MD, USA). The relative intensity was calibrated as a percentage, with the vehicle-sham group, which was designated as 100%.

4.6. Immunohistochemistry (IHC)

IHC was done to examine the effects of pretreated laminarin on IR-induced oxidative stress and neuroinflammation. Briefly, as described previously [45], the brain sections obtained at sham, 1 day and 5 days after IR were incubated with a solution of mouse anti-HNE (1:1000, Alexis Biochemicals, San Diego, CA, USA) for lipid peroxidation, a solution of sheep anti-SOD1 (1:1000, Calbiochem, La Jolla, CA, USA) and a solution of sheep anti-SOD2 (1:1000, Calbiochem, La Jolla, CA, USA) for antioxidants, a solution of rabbit anti-IL-1β (1:200, Santa Cruz Biotechnology, Santa Cruz, CA, USA) and a solution of rabbit anti-TNFα (1:1000, Abcam, Cambridge, MA, USA) for the pro-inflammatory response, and a solution of rabbit anti-IL-4 (1:200, Santa Cruz Biotechnology, Santa Cruz, CA, USA) and a solution of rabbit anti-IL-13 (1:200, Santa Cruz Biotechnology, Santa Cruz, CA, USA) for the anti-inflammatory response. These incubated sections were reacted with a solution of biotinylated goat anti-mouse, sheep, or rabbit IgG (1:200, Vector Laboratories Inc., Burlingame, CA, USA) as a secondary antibody and exposed to a solution of avidin–biotin complex (1:300, Vector Laboratories Inc., Burlingame, CA, USA). Finally, these immunoreacted sections were visualized by reacting with a solution of 3,3′-diaminobenzidine tetrahydrochloride (Sigma–Aldrich, St. Louis, MO, USA).

The immunoreactive structure of each HNE, SOD1, SOD2, IL-1β, TNFα, IL-4 and IL-13 was quantitatively analyzed as a relative immunoreactivity (RI). As previously described [45], in short, an image of each immunoreactive structure was captured with an Axio Imager 2 microscope (Carl Zeiss, Oberkochen, Germany) equipped with a digital camera. Each image was calibrated into an array of 512 × 512 pixels, and the immunoreactivity of each structure was evaluated on the basis of optical density (OD), which was obtained after the transformation of the mean gray level of each immunoreactive structure using a formula: OD = log (256/mean gray level). Finally, RI was calibrated as a percentage by using Adobe Photoshop (version 8.0, San Jose, CA, USA) and NIH Image software (1.59). The ratio of RI was calibrated as a percentage, with the vehicle-sham group designated as 100%.

4.7. Statistical Analysis

Data are presented as the means ± standard errors of the mean (SEM). All statistical analyses were performed using GraphPad Prism (version 5.0) (GraphPad Software, La Jolla, CA, USA). A multiple-sample comparison was applied to test the IR-related differences between the groups (two-way analysis of variance [ANOVA] and the Bonferroni's multiple comparison test as a post hoc test using the criterion of the least significant differences). Statistical significance was considered at $p < 0.05$.

Author Contributions: J.H.P., J.H.A., S.Y.C., and M.-H.W. were responsible for experimental design, data collection, and manuscript writing. T.-K.L., C.W.P., B.K., and D.W.K. performed the experiments and measurements, and J.-C.L., M.C.S., J.H.C., and C.-H.L. analyzed and interpreted data, and comments on the whole process of this study. All authors have read and agreed to the published version of the manuscript.

Funding: This research was funded by "Cooperative Research Program for Agriculture Science and Technology Development Rural Development Administration, Republic of Korea, grant number (Project No. PJ01321101)" and by "Basic Science Research Program through the National Research Foundation of Korea (NRF) funded by the Ministry of Education, grant number (2019R1A6A1A11036849)".

Conflicts of Interest: The authors declare that they have no competing interests.

References

1. Burad, J.; Bhakta, P.; George, J.; Kiruchennan, S. Development of acute ischemic stroke in a patient with acute respiratory distress syndrome (ARDS) resulting from H1N1 pneumonia. *Acta Anaesthesiol. Taiwanica* **2012**, *50*, 41–45. [CrossRef] [PubMed]
2. Kawai, K.; Nitecka, L.; Ruetzler, C.A.; Nagashima, G.; Joó, F.; Mies, G.; Nowak, T.S.; Saito, N.; Lohr, J.M.; Klatzo, I. Global Cerebral Ischemia Associated with Cardiac Arrest in the Rat: I. Dynamics of Early Neuronal Changes. *Br. J. Pharmacol.* **1992**, *12*, 238–249. [CrossRef] [PubMed]
3. Lee, J.-C.; Park, J.H.; Ahn, J.H.; Kim, I.H.; Cho, J.H.; Choi, J.H.; Yoo, K.-Y.; Lee, C.H.; Hwang, I.K.; Cho, J.H.; et al. New GABAergic Neurogenesis in the Hippocampal CA1 Region of a Gerbil Model of Long-Term Survival after Transient Cerebral Ischemic Injury. *Brain Pathol.* **2015**, *26*, 581–592. [CrossRef] [PubMed]
4. Von Kummer, R.; Bourquain, H.; Bastianello, S.; Bozzao, L.; Manelfe, C.; Meier, D.; Hacke, W. Early Prediction of Irreversible Brain Damage after Ischemic Stroke at CT. *Radiology* **2001**, *219*, 95–100. [CrossRef]
5. Thrift, A.G.; Cadilhac, D.A.; Thayabaranathan, T.; Howard, G.; Howard, V.J.; Rothwell, P.M.; Donnan, G.A. Global stroke statistics. *Int. J. Stroke* **2014**, *9*, 6–18. [CrossRef]
6. Harukuni, I.; Bhardwaj, A. Mechanisms of Brain Injury after Global Cerebral Ischemia. *Neurol. Clin.* **2006**, *24*, 1–21. [CrossRef]

7. Sugawara, T.; Lewén, A.; Noshita, N.; Gasche, Y.; Chan, P.H. Effects of Global Ischemia Duration on Neuronal, Astroglial, Oligodendroglial, and Microglial Reactions in the Vulnerable Hippocampal CA1 Subregion in Rats. *J. Neurotrauma* **2002**, *19*, 85–98. [CrossRef]
8. Iadecola, C.; Alexander, M. Cerebral ischemia and inflammation. *Curr. Opin. Neurol.* **2001**, *14*, 89–94. [CrossRef]
9. Saito, A.; Maier, C.M.; Narasimhan, P.; Nishi, T.; Song, Y.S.; Yu, F.; Liu, J.; Lee, Y.-S.; Nito, C.; Kamada, H.; et al. Oxidative Stress and Neuronal Death/Survival Signaling in Cerebral Ischemia. *Mol. Neurobiol.* **2005**, *31*, 105–116. [CrossRef]
10. Shichita, T.; Sakaguchi, R.; Suzuki, M.; Yoshimura, A. Post-Ischemic Inflammation in the Brain. *Front. Immunol.* **2012**, *3*, 132. [CrossRef]
11. Yang, S.-H.; Li, W. Targeting oxidative stress for the treatment of ischemic stroke: Upstream and downstream therapeutic strategies. *Brain Circ.* **2016**, *2*, 153–163. [CrossRef] [PubMed]
12. Peng, T.; Jiang, Y.; Farhan, M.; Lazarovici, P.; Chen, L.; Zheng, W. Anti-inflammatory Effects of Traditional Chinese Medicines on Preclinical in vivo Models of Brain Ischemia-Reperfusion-Injury: Prospects for Neuroprotective Drug Discovery and Therapy. *Front. Pharmacol.* **2019**, *10*, 204. [CrossRef] [PubMed]
13. Surgucheva, I.; Sharov, V.S.; Surguchov, A. γ-Synuclein: Seeding of α-Synuclein Aggregation and Transmission between Cells. *Biochemistry* **2012**, *51*, 4743–4754. [CrossRef] [PubMed]
14. Jin, X.; Wang, R.-H.; Wang, H.; Long, C.-L.; Wang, H. Brain protection against ischemic stroke using choline as a new molecular bypass treatment. *Acta Pharmacol. Sin.* **2015**, *36*, 1416–1425. [CrossRef]
15. Zhang, H.; Park, J.H.; Maharjan, S.; Park, J.A.; Choi, K.-S.; Park, H.; Jeong, Y.; Ahn, J.H.; Kim, I.H.; Lee, J.-C.; et al. Sac-1004, a vascular leakage blocker, reduces cerebral ischemia—Reperfusion injury by suppressing blood–brain barrier disruption and inflammation. *J. Neuroinflamm.* **2017**, *14*, 122. [CrossRef]
16. Zhang, W.; Song, J.; Yan, R.; Li, L.; Xiao, Z.-Y.; Zhou, W.-X.; Wang, Z.-Z.; Xiao, W.; Du, G.-H. Diterpene ginkgolides protect against cerebral ischemia/reperfusion damage in rats by activating Nrf2 and CREB through PI3K/Akt signaling. *Acta Pharmacol. Sin.* **2018**, *39*, 1259–1272. [CrossRef]
17. Benjamin, E.J.; Blaha, M.J.; Chiuve, S.E.; Cushman, M.; Das, S.R.; Deo, R.; De Ferranti, S.D.; Floyd, J.; Fornage, M.; Gillespie, C.; et al. Heart Disease and Stroke Statistics—2017 Update: A Report From the American Heart Association. *Circulation* **2017**, *135*, e146–e603. [CrossRef]
18. Zhou, Z.; Ji, X.; Zhang, L.; Liu, R.; Liu, Y.; Song, J.; Dong, H.; Jia, Y. Potential targets for protecting against hippocampal cell apoptosis after transient cerebral ischemia-reperfusion injury in aged rats. *Neural Regen. Res.* **2014**, *9*, 1122–1128. [CrossRef]
19. Saucier, D.M.; Yager, J.Y.; Armstrong, E.A.; Keller, A.; Shultz, S.R. Enriched environment and the effect of age on ischemic brain damage. *Brain Res.* **2007**, *1170*, 31–38. [CrossRef]
20. Xu, K.; Puchowicz, M.A.; Sun, X.; Lamanna, J.C. Mitochondrial Dysfunction in Aging Rat Brain Following Transient Global Ischemia. *Single Mol. Single Cell Seq.* **2008**, *614*, 379–386. [CrossRef]
21. Davis, M.; Mendelow, A.D.; Perry, R.H.; Chambers, I.; James, O.F.W. Experimental Stroke and Neuroprotection in the Aging Rat Brain. *Stroke* **1995**, *26*, 1072–1078. [CrossRef] [PubMed]
22. Pohl, F.; Kong-Thoo-Lin, P. The Potential Use of Plant Natural Products and Plant Extracts with Antioxidant Properties for the Prevention/Treatment of Neurodegenerative Diseases: In Vitro, In Vivo and Clinical Trials. *Molecule* **2018**, *23*, 3283. [CrossRef] [PubMed]
23. Wu, P.-F.; Zhang, Z.; Wang, F.; Chen, J.-G. Natural compounds from traditional medicinal herbs in the treatment of cerebral ischemia/reperfusion injury. *Acta Pharmacol. Sin.* **2010**, *31*, 1523–1531. [CrossRef] [PubMed]
24. Ahn, J.H.; Shin, M.C.; Kim, D.W.; Kim, H.; Song, M.; Lee, T.-K.; Lee, J.-C.; Kim, H.; Cho, J.H.; Kim, Y.-M.; et al. Antioxidant Properties of Fucoidan Alleviate Acceleration and Exacerbation of Hippocampal Neuronal Death Following Transient Global Cerebral Ischemia in High-Fat Diet-Induced Obese Gerbils. *Int. J. Mol. Sci.* **2019**, *20*, 554. [CrossRef]
25. Che, N.; Ma, Y.; Xin, Y. Protective Role of Fucoidan in Cerebral Ischemia-Reperfusion Injury through Inhibition of MAPK Signaling Pathway. *Biomol. Ther.* **2016**, *25*, 272–278. [CrossRef]
26. Kang, G.H.; Yan, B.C.; Cho, G.-S.; Kim, W.-K.; Lee, C.H.; Cho, J.H.; Kim, M.; Kang, I.-J.; Won, M.-H.; Lee, J.-C. Neuroprotective effect of fucoidin on lipopolysaccharide accelerated cerebral ischemic injury through inhibition of cytokine expression and neutrophil infiltration. *J. Neurol. Sci.* **2012**, *318*, 25–30. [CrossRef]

27. Kim, H.; Ahn, J.H.; Song, M.; Kim, D.W.; Lee, T.-K.; Lee, J.-C.; Kim, Y.-M.; Kim, J.-D.; Cho, J.H.; Hwang, I.K.; et al. Pretreated fucoidan confers neuroprotection against transient global cerebral ischemic injury in the gerbil hippocampal CA1 area via reducing of glial cell activation and oxidative stress. *Biomed. Pharmacother.* **2019**, *109*, 1718–1727. [CrossRef]
28. Lee, T.-K.; Ahn, J.H.; Park, C.; Kim, B.; Park, Y.; Lee, J.-C.; Park, J.H.; Yang, G.; Shin, M.; Cho, J.; et al. Pre-Treatment with Laminarin Protects Hippocampal CA1 Pyramidal Neurons and Attenuates Reactive Gliosis Following Transient Forebrain Ischemia in Gerbils. *Mar. Drugs* **2020**, *18*, 52. [CrossRef]
29. Kim, K.-H.; Kim, Y.-W.; Kim, H.B.; Lee, B.J.; Lee, D.S. Anti-apoptotic Activity of Laminarin Polysaccharides and their Enzymatically Hydrolyzed Oligosaccharides from Laminaria japonica. *Biotechnol. Lett.* **2006**, *28*, 439–446. [CrossRef]
30. Cheng, D.; Liang, B.; Li, M.; Jin, M. Influence of Laminarin polysaccharides on oxidative damage. *Int. J. Biol. Macromol.* **2011**, *48*, 63–66. [CrossRef]
31. Neyrinck, A.M.; Mouson, A.; Delzenne, N.M. Dietary supplementation with laminarin, a fermentable marine β (1–3) glucan, protects against hepatotoxicity induced by LPS in rat by modulating immune response in the hepatic tissue. *Int. Immunopharmacol.* **2007**, *7*, 1497–1506. [CrossRef] [PubMed]
32. Song, K.; Xu, L.; Zhang, W.; Cai, Y.; Jang, B.; Oh, J.; Jin, J.-O. Laminarin promotes anti-cancer immunity by the maturation of dendritic cells. *Oncotarget* **2017**, *8*, 38554–38567. [CrossRef] [PubMed]
33. Globus, M.Y.; Busto, R.; Martinez, E.; Valdés, I.; Dietrich, W.D.; Ginsberg, M.D. Comparative effect of transient global ischemia on extracellular levels of glutamate, glycine, and gamma-aminobutyric acid in vulnerable and nonvulnerable brain regions in the rat. *J. Neurochem.* **1991**, *57*, 470–478. [CrossRef] [PubMed]
34. Pulsinelli, W.A.; Brierley, J.B.; Plum, F. Temporal profile of neuronal damage in a model of transient forebrain ischemia. *Ann. Neurol.* **1982**, *11*, 491–498. [CrossRef]
35. Petito, C.K.; Feldmann, E.; Pulsinelli, W.A.; Plum, F. Delayed hippocampal damage in humans following cardiorespiratory arrest. *Neurology* **1987**, *37*, 1281. [CrossRef]
36. Gemma, C.; Vila, J.; Bachstetter, A.; Bickford, P.C. *Oxidative Stress and the Aging Brain: From Theory to Prevention*; Riddle, D.R., Ed.; Brain Aging: Boca Raton, FL, USA, 2007.
37. Sparkman, N.L.; Johnson, R. Neuroinflammation associated with aging sensitizes the brain to the effects of infection or stress. *Neuroimmunomodulation* **2008**, *15*, 323–330. [CrossRef]
38. Olmez, I.; Ozyurt, H. Reactive oxygen species and ischemic cerebrovascular disease. *Neurochem. Int.* **2012**, *60*, 208–212. [CrossRef]
39. Godinho, J.; De Sá-Nakanishi, A.B.; Moreira, L.S.; De Oliveira, R.M.W.; Huzita, C.H.; Mello, J.C.P.; Da Silva, A.O.F.; Nakamura, C.V.; Previdelli, I.S.; Ribeiro, M.H.D.M.; et al. Ethyl-acetate fraction of Trichilia catigua protects against oxidative stress and neuroinflammation after cerebral ischemia/reperfusion. *J. Ethnopharmacol.* **2018**, *221*, 109–118. [CrossRef]
40. Viswanatha, G.L.; Shylaja, H.; Mohan, C. Alleviation of transient global ischemia/reperfusion-induced brain injury in rats with 1,2,3,4,6-penta-O-galloyl-β-d-glucopyranose isolated from Mangifera indica. *Eur. J. Pharmacol.* **2013**, *720*, 286–293. [CrossRef]
41. He, L.; He, T.; Farrar, S.; Ji, L.; Liu, T.; Ma, X. Antioxidants Maintain Cellular Redox Homeostasis by Elimination of Reactive Oxygen Species. *Cell. Physiol. Biochem.* **2017**, *44*, 532–553. [CrossRef]
42. Davis, S.; Pennypacker, K.R. Targeting antioxidant enzyme expression as a therapeutic strategy for ischemic stroke. *Neurochem. Int.* **2016**, *107*, 23–32. [CrossRef] [PubMed]
43. Yang, M.-S.; Park, E.J.; Sohn, S.; Kwon, H.J.; Shin, W.-H.; Pyo, H.K.; Jin, B.; Choi, K.; Jou, I.; Joe, E.-H. Interleukin-13 and -4 induce death of activated microglia. *Glia* **2002**, *38*, 273–280. [CrossRef] [PubMed]
44. Troup, G.; Smith, G.; Walford, R. Life span, chronologic disease patterns, and age-related changes in relative spleen weights for the mongolian gerbil (Meriones unguiculatus). *Exp. Gerontol.* **1969**, *4*, 139–143. [CrossRef]
45. Park, J.H.; Ahn, J.H.; Song, M.; Kim, H.; Park, C.; Park, Y.; Lee, T.-K.; Lee, J.-C.; Kim, D.W.; Lee, C.-H.; et al. A 2-Min Transient Ischemia Confers Cerebral Ischemic Tolerance in Non-Obese Gerbils, but Results in Neuronal Death in Obese Gerbils by Increasing Abnormal mTOR Activation-Mediated Oxidative Stress and Neuroinflammation. *Cells* **2019**, *8*, 1126. [CrossRef] [PubMed]
46. Song, M.; Ahn, J.H.; Kim, H.; Kim, D.W.; Lee, T.-K.; Lee, J.-C.; Kim, Y.-M.; Lee, C.-H.; Hwang, I.K.; Yan, B.C.; et al. Chronic high-fat diet-induced obesity in gerbils increases pro-inflammatory cytokines and mTOR activation, and elicits neuronal death in the striatum following brief transient ischemia. *Neurochem. Int.* **2018**, *121*, 75–85. [CrossRef] [PubMed]

47. Lee, J.C.; Park, J.H.; Kim, I.H.; Cho, G.S.; Ahn, J.H.; Tae, H.J.; Choi, S.Y.; Cho, J.H.; Kim, D.W.; Kwon, Y.G.; et al. Neuroprotection of ischemic preconditioning is mediated by thioredoxin 2 in the hippocampal CA1 region following a subsequent transient cerebral ischemia. *Brain Pathol.* **2017**, *27*, 276–291. [CrossRef] [PubMed]
48. Radtke-Schuller, S.; Schuller, G.; Angenstein, F.; Grosser, O.S.; Goldschmidt, J.; Budinger, E. Brain atlas of the Mongolian gerbil (Meriones unguiculatus) in CT/MRI-aided stereotaxic coordinates. *Brain Struct. Funct.* **2016**, *221*, 1–272. [CrossRef]

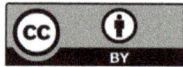

© 2020 by the authors. Licensee MDPI, Basel, Switzerland. This article is an open access article distributed under the terms and conditions of the Creative Commons Attribution (CC BY) license (http://creativecommons.org/licenses/by/4.0/).

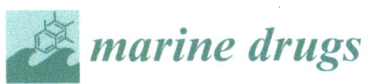

Article

Anti-Inflammatory and Protein Tyrosine Phosphatase 1B Inhibitory Metabolites from the Antarctic Marine-Derived Fungal Strain *Penicillium glabrum* SF-7123

Tran Minh Ha [1,†], Dong-Cheol Kim [1,†], Jae Hak Sohn [2], Joung Han Yim [3,*] and Hyuncheol Oh [1,*]

1. Institute of Pharmaceutical Research and Development, College of Pharmacy, Wonkwang University, Iksan 54538, Korea; minhha19@outlook.com (T.M.H.); kimman07@hanmail.net (D.-C.K.)
2. College of Medical and Life Sciences, Silla University, Busan 46958, Korea; jhsohn@silla.ac.kr
3. Korea Polar Research Institute, KORDI, 7-50 Songdo-dong, Yeonsu-gu, Incheon 21990, Korea
* Correspondence: jhyim@kopri.re.kr (J.H.Y.); hoh@wku.ac.kr (H.O.);
  Tel.: +82-32-760-5540 (J.H.Y.); +82-63-850-6815 (H.O.)
† These authors contributed equally.

Received: 22 April 2020; Accepted: 6 May 2020; Published: 9 May 2020

Abstract: A chemical investigation of the marine-derived fungal strain *Penicillium glabrum* (SF-7123) revealed a new citromycetin (polyketide) derivative (**1**) and four known secondary fungal metabolites, i.e, neuchromenin (**2**), asterric acid (**3**), myxotrichin C (**4**), and deoxyfunicone (**5**). The structures of these metabolites were identified primarily by extensive analysis of their spectroscopic data, including NMR and MS data. Results from the initial screening of anti-inflammatory effects showed that **2**, **4**, and **5** possessed inhibitory activity against the excessive production of nitric oxide (NO) in lipopolysaccharide (LPS)-stimulated BV2 microglial cells, with IC_{50} values of 2.7 µM, 28.1 µM, and 10.6 µM, respectively. Compounds **2**, **4**, and **5** also inhibited the excessive production of NO, with IC_{50} values of 4.7 µM, 41.5 µM, and 40.1 µM, respectively, in LPS-stimulated RAW264.7 macrophage cells. In addition, these compounds inhibited LPS-induced overproduction of prostaglandin E_2 in both cellular models. Further investigation of the most active compound (**2**) revealed that these anti-inflammatory effects were associated with a suppressive effect on the over-expression of inducible nitric oxide synthase and cyclooxygenase-2. Finally, we showed that the anti-inflammatory effects of compound **2** were mediated via the downregulation of inflammation-related pathways such as those dependent on nuclear factor kappa B and p38 mitogen-activated protein kinase in LPS-stimulated BV2 and RAW264.7 cells. In the evaluation of the inhibitory effects of the isolated compounds on protein tyrosine phosphate 1B (PTP1B) activity, compound **4** was identified as a noncompetitive inhibitor of PTP1B, with an IC_{50} value of 19.2 µM, and compound **5** was shown to inhibit the activity of PTP1B, with an IC_{50} value of 24.3 µM, by binding to the active site of the enzyme. Taken together, this study demonstrates the potential value of marine-derived fungal isolates as a bioresource for bioactive compounds.

Keywords: marine-derived fungi; anti-inflammation; anti-neuroinflammation; PTP1B

1. Introduction

Marine-derived fungi have been suggested as a unique source of bioactive secondary metabolites [1,2]. In recent years, research interest in marine-derived fungi as a valuable resource of bioactive compounds has significantly increased, resulting in the exploration of a variety of novel metabolites, consisting of polyketides (40%), alkaloids (20%), peptides (15%), terpenoids (15%), prenylated polyketides (7%), as well as shikimates (2%) and lipids (1%) [3]. The chemical study of the ethyl acetate (EtOAc) extract obtained from the culture of the marine-derived fungal strain *Penicillium glabrum* (SF-7123) has been the focus of our continuing efforts to find bioactive secondary metabolites from marine-derived fungal strains collected in Antarctic area. The fungal strain SF-7123 was cultured on Petri agar plates (containing 3% NaCl) at 25 °C for three weeks. The culture media were extracted with EtOAc, and the filtered extracts were then concentrated in vacuo to provide a crude extract. A combination of chromatographic methods was employed to yield a new citromycetin derivative (**1**) and four known secondary metabolites (**2–5**) from the crude extract (Figure 1).

The chemical investigation of the extract from the fungal strain SF-7123 utilized a bioassay system for the evaluation of anti-inflammatory effects in cellular models to detect the bioactive fractions and pure fungal metabolites from the crude extract. Inflammation is recognized as a vital reaction of the body to injury or infection. Macrophages and microglia (the resident macrophage-like cells of the central nervous system) have been repeatedly reported to exert a key role in the immune system [4,5]. They are activated in response to various stimuli and lead to phagocytosis of damaged macrophages and neuronal cells to protect tissues and prevent damage to the brain and body. However, their sustained activation leads to the release of pro-inflammatory mediators such as inducible nitric oxide synthase (iNOS), cyclooxygenase-2 (COX-2), NO, and prostaglandin E_2 (PGE_2), as well as of pro-inflammatory cytokines, including tumor necrosis factor (TNF)-α, interleukin (IL)-1β, IL-6, and IL-12. These mediators and cytokines are known to be detrimental to cells or tissues and to cause various inflammatory diseases, including inflammatory bowel disease, Alzheimer's disease, Parkinson's disease, and multiple sclerosis [6–9]. Therefore, controlling the production of pro-inflammatory mediators/cytokines could be regarded as a reasonable target for the prevention and/or treatment of inflammatory diseases. For many years, the RAW264.7 cell line (Abelson murine leukemia virus-transformed macrophage cells derived from male BALB/c mice) has been widely accepted as an in vitro model to investigate cellular inflammation responses. Likewise, BV2 cells (raf/myc-immortalized murine microglia) have been frequently employed to model the reactions of microglia in vivo.

To gain further information with respect to the biological effects of the fungal metabolites isolated in this study, an enzymatic assay system to evaluate the inhibitory effects on protein tyrosine phosphatase 1B (PTP1B) was also employed throughout the study. PTP1B is a major negative regulator of insulin and leptin signaling pathways. It has been reported that PTP1B is related to inflammation in many tissues, such as hypothalamus and lungs, and plays an important role in lipopolysaccharide (LPS)-induced activation of microglia and macrophages [10,11]. Furthermore, many studies have indicated that PTP1B expression is increased under many pathophysiological conditions such as inflammation, cancer, and diabetes, suggesting novel therapeutic implications for these PTP1B inhibitors in the treatment of such diseases [12].

2. Results and Discussion

2.1. Isolation and Structure Determination of Compounds 1–5

Compound 1 was isolated as an amorphous powder, optically active, with an $[\alpha]_D^{20}$ value of −344.63 (c 0.48, CH_3OH). The HRESIMS (Supplementary Materials, Figure S1) of **1** showed an ion peak at m/z 263.0911 [M + H]$^+$ (calcd for $C_{14}H_{15}O_5$, 263.0919), determining the molecular formula $C_{14}H_{14}O_5$. The ^{1}H NMR spectrum of **1** (Table 1, Figure S2) disclosed the typical signals for two aromatic protons at δ_H 6.34 (1H, s, H-7) and 7.06 (1H, s, H-10), a singlet peak at δ_H 3.83 (3H, H-12) for methoxy protons, and a signal for methyl protons at δ_H 1.55 (3H, d, J = 6.4, H-11). In addition, there were three downfield-shifted signals corresponding to an oxymethine proton at δ_H 4.71 (1H, m, H-2) and oxymethylene protons at δ_H 4.73 (1H, d, J = 12.0, H-5a) and δ_H 5.03 (1H, d, J = 12.0, H-5b). The remaining signal at δ_H 2.53 (2H, m, H-3) was assigned to a methylene proton. The ^{13}C NMR spectra (Figure S3) of **1** displayed 14 carbons, including 9 sp^2 signals assigned to a carbonyl group at δ_C 191.0 (C-4), and two aromatic methine carbons at δ_C 104.8 (C-7) and δ_C 108.9 (C-10). In addition, six sp^2 quaternary carbon signals at δ_C 102.4 (C-4a), 156.3 (C-6a), 154.5 (C-8), 144.8 (C-9), 107.9 (C-10a), and 165.7 (C-10b) were present in the spectrum. The two oxygenated carbons at δ_C 77.3 and δ_C 64.1

were identified as a methine (C-2) and a methylene (C-5), respectively. The ^{13}C NMR spectra of **1** also displayed signals for a methoxy group at δ_C 57.0 (C-12), a methylene carbon at δ_C 43.5 (C-3), and a methyl group at δ_C 20.6 (C-11). A literature review revealed that the ^{1}H and ^{13}C NMR data of **1** were similar to those reported for neuchromenin [13,14], indicating close structural similarity between the two compounds, except for the presence of a methoxy group in **1**. A detailed analysis of the COSY and HMBC spectra of **1** (Table 1, Figures S4 and S5) confirmed the planar structure of **1** as a derivative of neuchromenin with the replacement of the hydroxy group by a methoxy group attached to C-9. This was supported by the observation of an HMBC correlation from 9-OCH$_3$ to C-9. Consequently, on the basis of this evidence, the structure of compound **1** was determined as shown in Figure 1 and named 9-*O*-methylneuchromenin.

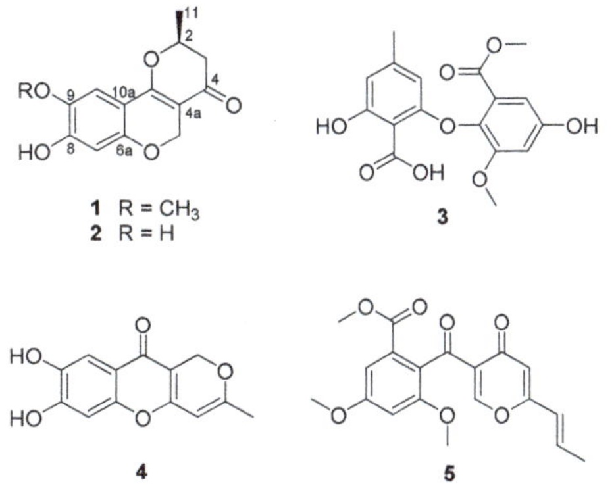

Figure 1. Chemical structures of compounds **1–5**.

Table 1. NMR data of 9-*O*-methylneuchromenin (**1**).

Position	δ_C [a,b]	δ_H [a,c] (mult, J in Hz)	HMBC
2	77.3	4.72 (m)	
3	43.5	2.53 (m)	2, 4, 11
4	191.0	-	-
4a	102.4	-	-
5	64.1	5.03 (d, 12.0), 4.73 (d, 12.0)	4, 4a, 6a, 10b
6a	156.3	-	-
7	104.8	6.34 (s)	6a, 8, 9, 10, 10b
8	154.5	-	-
9	144.8	-	-
10	108.9	7.06 (s)	6a, 8, 9, 10, 10b
10a	107.9	-	
10b	165.7	-	-
11	20.6	1.55 (d, 6.4)	2, 3, 4
12	57.0	3.83 (s)	9

[a] Recorded in CD$_3$OD, [b] 100 MHz, [c] 400 MHz.

The NMR data of compound **2** (Figure S6) were almost identical to those of **1**, indicating a pyranchromene skeleton typical of citromycetin analogues. A close inspection of the ^{1}H and ^{13}C NMR data of compound **2** and their comparison with those found in the literature eventually led to the assignment of the structure of neuchromenin, which has been isolated from the culture broth of *Eupenicillium javanicum* var. *meloforme* PF1181. Neuchromenin reportedly induced neurite outgrowth in PC12 pheochromocytoma cells in a rat model [13]. The absolute configuration of naturally occurring neuchromenin was previously determined to be *S*-configuration via the synthetic study of the enantiomers of neuchromenin [14]. Close similarities with data reported in the literature are found for the NMR data and the well-matched specific rotation value of **2** [15], suggesting that compound **2** must have the same absolute configuration at C-2 as that of (−)-neuchromenin. Accordingly, the absolute configuration of **1** was suggested to be analogous to that of **2**, because these fungal metabolites were produced by the same fungal strain.

The structures of the remaining compounds were also determined based on the analysis of their NMR (Figures S7–S9) and MS data, along with a comparison with previously published data in the literature. A diphenyl ether was isolated in this study, which was identified as asterric acid (**3**), known as an endothelin binding inhibitor [16,17]. Compound **4** was identified as a citromycetin derivative, i.e., myxotrichin C [18]. There are no previous reports on the biological effects of this metabolite. The structure of compound **5** was elucidated and found to be deoxyfunicone, which could be classified as a phenolic polyketide and a funicone analogue [19]; it was described as an HIV-1-integrase inhibitor [20].

2.2. Effects of Secondary Metabolites Isolated from SF-7123 on the Production of Pro-Inflammatory Mediators

LPS is a major cell wall component of Gram-negative bacteria. LPS is an intensive stimulator of macrophages and microglia, and thus treatment of these cells with LPS is frequently employed in research related to the inflammatory phenomenon [21,22]. In the current study, all the isolated compounds (**1–5**) were investigated for their anti-neuroinflammatory and anti-inflammatory effects by examining their effects on the overproduction of NO and PGE_2 in LPS-stimulated BV2 microglia and RAW264.7 macrophage cells. LPS stimulation increased the production of NO and PGE_2 in both cell lines. Pre-treatment with **2**, **4**, and **5** attenuated these responses, with different IC_{50} values as shown in Table 2. Compounds **1** and **3** did not significantly affect to the alteration of NO production at 80.0 μM. On the basis of the IC_{50} values of **1** and **2** and their respective structures, we reasoned that the replacement of the hydroxy group at position C-9 in neuchromenin (**2**) by a methoxy group would decrease this inhibitory effect significantly. The most active compound in the assay was identified to be **2**. Thus, this compound was selected to further examine the anti-inflammatory effect and to reveal its underlying mechanisms. Compound **2** effectively decreased the mRNA over-expressions of IL-1β, TNF-α, IL-6, and IL-12 in LPS-stimulated BV2 and RAW264.7 cells (Figure 2) when the cells were activated with LPS (1 μg/mL) for 12 h. Moreover, compound **2** attenuated the protein expression of iNOS and COX-2 in a dose-dependent manner in LPS-stimulated BV2 cells (Figure 3A). In LPS-stimulated RAW264.7 cells, compound **2** dose-dependently attenuated the protein expression of COX-2, and a significant attenuation of iNOS expression was observed at a concentration of 4.0 μM (Figure 3B). To confirm that the observed anti-inflammatory effects did not arise from their cytotoxicity, the MTT assay was conducted in the presence of the compounds tested, and the results showed that compounds **1–5** were not cytotoxic to these cells at doses up to 80.0 μM (data not shown).

Table 2. Inhibitory effects (IC_{50} = μM) of compounds **1–5** on the overproduction of NO and prostaglandin E_2 (PGE_2) in lipopolysaccharide (LPS)-stimulated cells.

Compounds	NO Inhibitory Effects [a]		PGE_2 Inhibitory Effects [a]	
	BV2 Cells	RAW264.7 Cells	BV2 Cells	RAW264.7 Cells
1	>80	>80	>80	50.2 ± 2.5
2	2.7 ± 0.1	4.7 ± 0.2	3.2 ± 0.2	4.1 ± 0.1
3	>80	>80	>80	53.4 ± 2.7
4	28.1 ± 1.4	41.5 ± 2.1	25.2 ± 1.3	30.0 ± 1.5
5	10.6 ± 0.5	40.1 ± 2.0	32.3 ± 1.6	>80

[a] Values present mean ± SD of triplicate experiments.

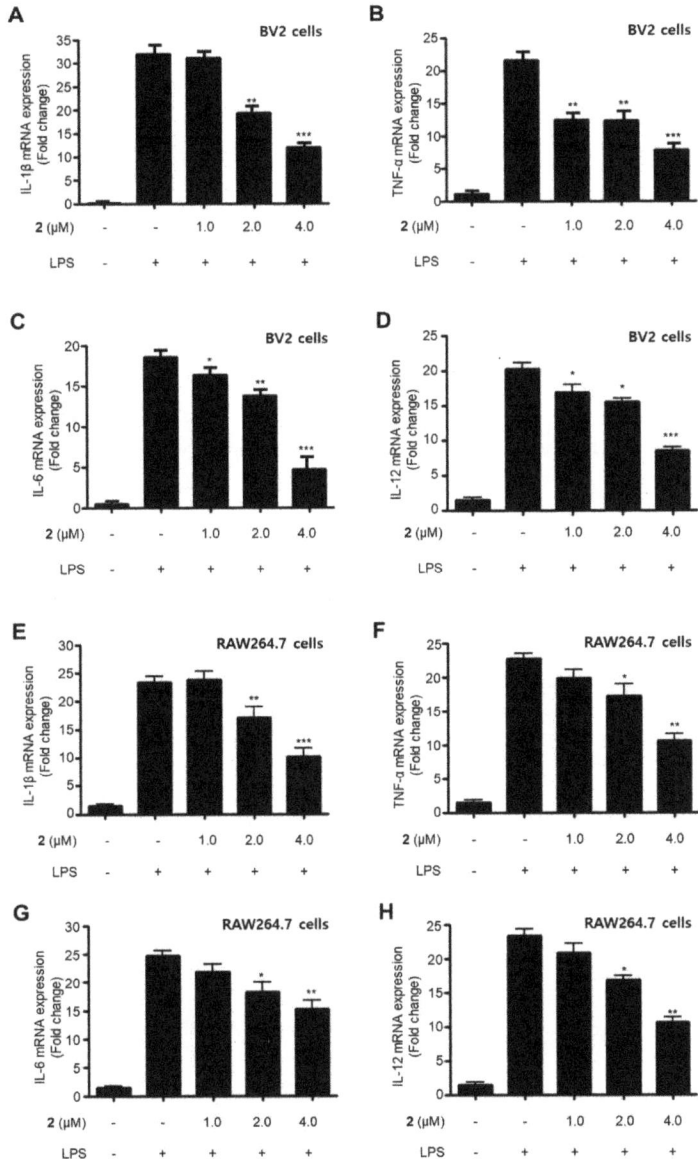

Figure 2. Suppressive effects of compound **2** on the mRNA expression of pro-inflammatory cytokines IL-1β (**A,E**), TNF-α (**B,F**), IL-6 (**C,G**), and IL-12 (**D,H**) in LPS-stimulated BV2 and RAW264.7 cells. After pre-treatment for 3 h with the indicated concentrations of compound **2**, the cells were stimulated for 12 h with LPS (1 μg/mL). Data represent the mean values of three experiments ± SD (* $p < 0.05$; ** $p < 0.01$; *** $p < 0.001$) compared to the LPS-treated group.

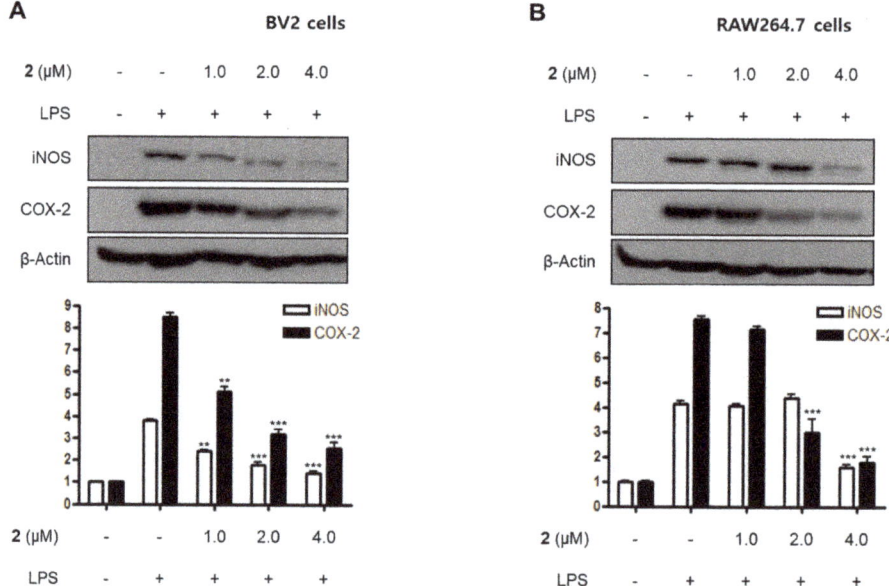

Figure 3. Effects of compound **2** on the protein expression of inducible nitric oxide synthase (iNOS) and cyclooxygenase-2 (COX-2) in LPS-induced BV2 (**A**) and RAW264.7 cells (**B**). Cells were pre-treated with compound **2** (1.0, 2.0, and 4.0 μM) for 3 h and stimulated with LPS (1 μg/mL) for 24 h. The representative blots of three independent analyses for iNOS and COX-2 expression are shown. Band intensity was quantified by densitometry and normalized to β-actin (** $p < 0.01$; *** $p < 0.001$) compared to the LPS-treated group.

2.3. Effect of Compound 2 on NF-κB and Mitogen-Activated Protein Kinase (MAPK) Pathways

Nuclear factor-kappa B (NF-κB) and MAPK are essential for the regulation of pro-inflammatory mediators and pro-inflammatory cytokines. Therefore, the pathways they regulate play a vital role in the inflammatory reaction. NF-κB is a transcription factor normally kept in the cytoplasm by inhibitor kappa B-α (IκB-α). Inflammatory stimulants such as LPS induce IκBs phosphorylation, which leads to the release of an NF-κB dimer (p50 and p65) that translocate into the nucleus, resulting in the transcription of inflammatory genes such iNOS, COX-2, NO, PGE_2, TNF-α, IL-1β, IL-6, and IL-12 [23–25]. Therefore, we examined the effects of compound **2** on the LPS-stimulated upregulation of the NF-κB pathway in BV2 and RAW264.7 cells. Immunoblotting assays revealed that compound **2** suppressed the activation of the NF-κB pathway in cells that were stimulated with LPS. For example, compound **2** reversed the phosphorylation and degradation of IκB-α (Figure 4A,B) and blocked the translocation of the NF-κB dimer (p50 and p65) into the nucleus (Figure 4C–F). Furthermore, compound **2** decreased the DNA binding activity of the p65 subunit (Figure 4G,H) in LPS-stimulated BV2 and RAW264.7 cells.

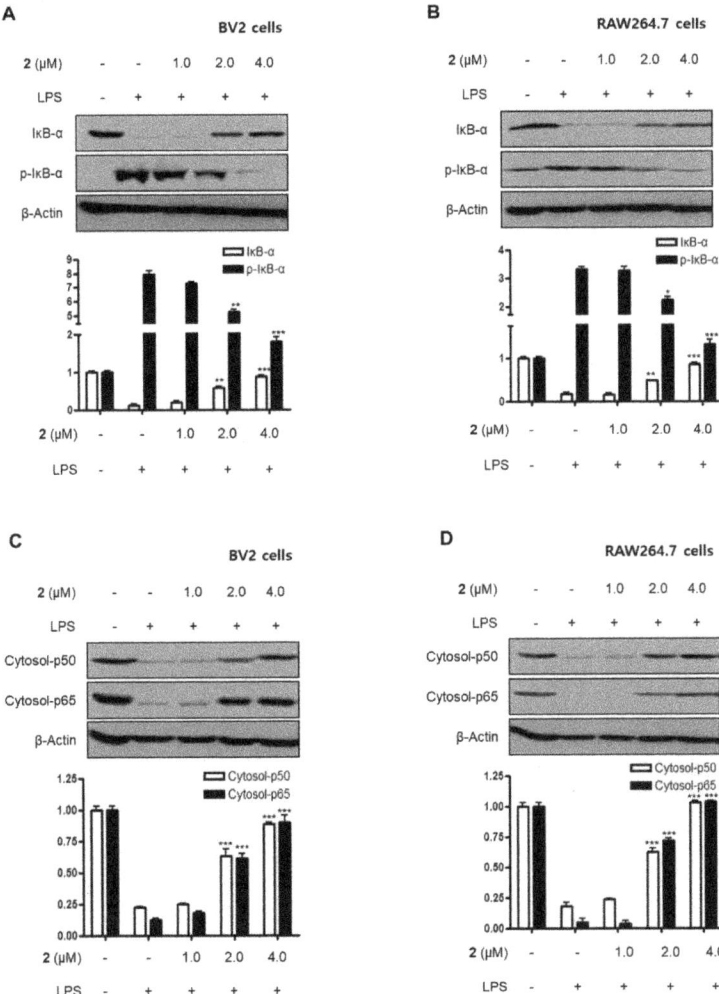

Figure 4. *Cont.*

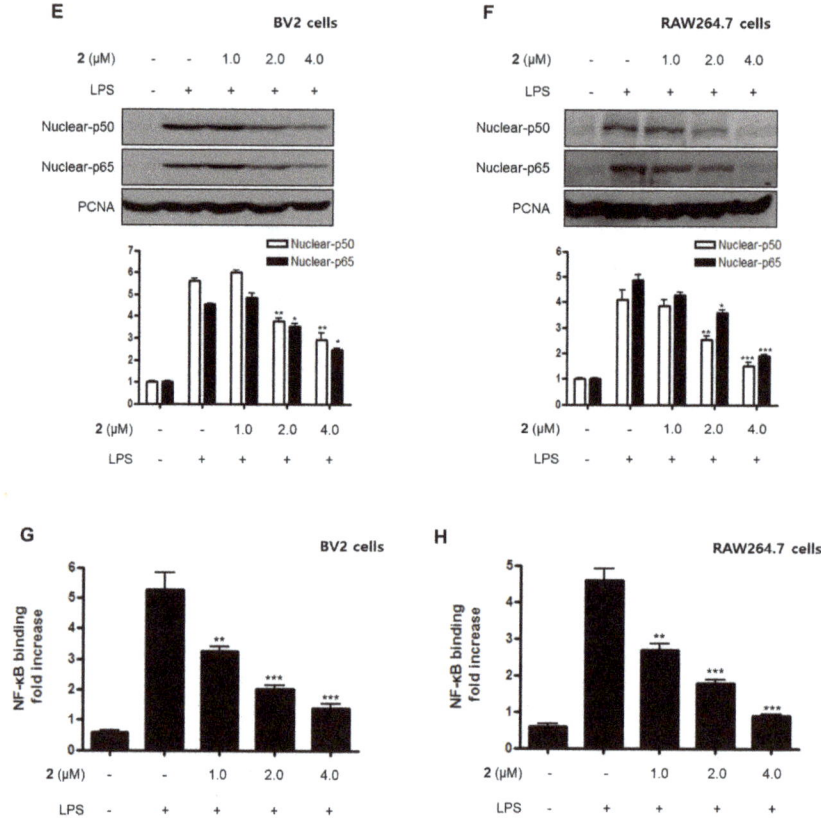

Figure 4. Effect of compound **2** on the activation of the NF-κB pathway in LPS-induced BV2 and RAW264.7 cells. After pre-treatment with compound **2** (1.0, 2.0, and 4.0 μM) for 3 h, the cells were stimulated with LPS for 1 h. (**A–F**) Proteins were obtained, and specific anti-IκB-α, anti-p- IκB-α, anti-p65, and anti-p50 antibodies were employed for western blot analysis. Representative blots of three independent experiments are shown. Band intensity was quantified by densitometry and normalized to β-actin for the cytoplasmic fraction and to proliferating cell nuclear antigen (PCNA) for the nuclear fraction. (**G, H**) NF-κB binding activity in the nuclear fraction was determined using an NF-κB ELISA kit by Active Motif (* $p < 0.05$; ** $p < 0.01$; *** $p < 0.001$) and then compared to that of the LPS-treated group.

MAPKs have been reported to play a critical role in a variety of cellular conditions such as cell death, cell growth, differentiation, proliferation, and immune responses [26,27]. MAPKs consist of three major signaling kinases, i.e., extracellular signal-regulated kinases 1 and 2 (ERK1/ERK2), c-Jun N-terminal kinases (JNKs), and p38 MAPK. Specifically, p38 MAPK is one of the MAPKs that regulate the inflammatory responses and is considered a therapeutic target for anti-inflammatory treatments. In this investigation, we examined the effects of compound **2** on LPS-stimulated activation of MAPKs in BV2 and RAW264.7 cells. When the cells were stimulated with LPS for 1 h, the phosphorylation levels of MAPKs were significantly upregulated. However, pre-treatment with compound **2** inhibited LPS-induced p38 MAPK phosphorylation in BV2 and RAW264.7 cells, whereas the increased phosphorylation levels of ERK and JNK MAPKs were unchanged (Figure 5). On the basis of these results, it was postulated that compound **2** exhibited anti-inflammatory and anti-neuroinflammatory effects via the suppression of the activation of NF-κB and p38 MAPK pathways.

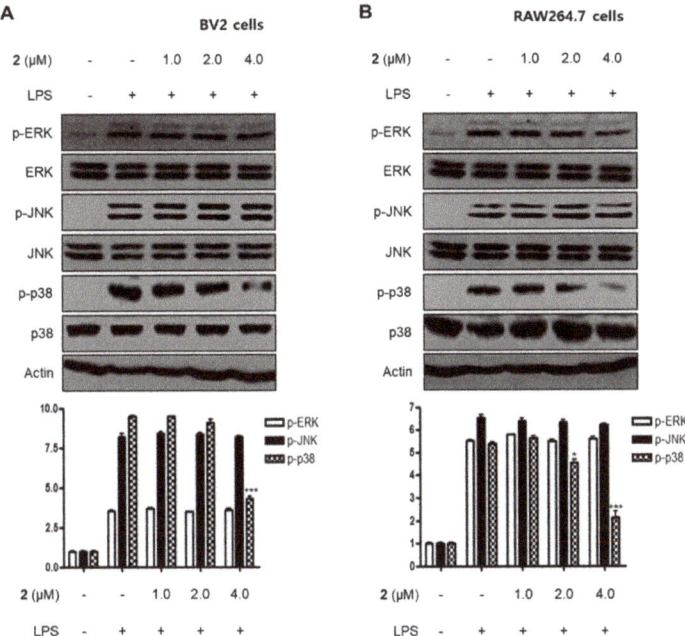

Figure 5. Effect of compound **2** on the activation of MAPK pathways in LPS-induced BV2 (**A**) and RAW264.7 cells (**B**). After pre-treatment with compound **2** (1.0, 2.0, and 4.0 μM) for 3 h, the cells were stimulated with LPS for 1 h. Western blot analysis was performed to determine the phosphorylated levels of extracellular signal-regulated kinases (ERK) (p-ERK), c-Jun N-terminal kinases (JNK) (p-JNK), and p38 MAPK (p-p38 MAPK). Representative blots of three independent experiments are shown. Band intensity was quantified by densitometry and normalized to β-actin. * $p < 0.05$; *** $p < 0.001$ as compared to the LPS-treated group.

2.4. PTP1B Inhibitory Effects of the Isolated Metabolites **1–5**

In addition to the investigation of the anti-inflammatory and anti-neuroinflammatory effects of the isolated metabolites in cellular models, this study attempted to assess the inhibitory effect of the isolated compounds against PTP1B activity. In this enzymatic assay, a known phosphatase inhibitor, ursolic acid, was used as a positive control, and *p*-nitrophenol phosphate (*p*NPP) was used as an enzyme substrate [28,29]. When compounds **1–5** at 50 μM concentration were incubated with PTP1B in the presence of the substrate, compounds **4** and **5** were shown to significantly inhibit the activity of PTP1B, whereas the inhibitory activity of compounds **1–3** was less pronounced. Furthermore, the inhibitory effects of compounds **4** and **5** were concentration-dependent, and their IC$_{50}$ values were determined to be 19.2 μM and 24.3 μM, respectively (Table 3).

Table 3. Inhibitory effects of compounds **1–5** on protein tyrosine phosphatase 1B (PTP1B).

Compounds	Inhibitory Effects on PTP1B [a]
1	45.7% [b]
2	37.8% [b]
3	13.7% [b]
4	19.2 ± 1.0
5	24.3 ± 1.2
Ursolic acid [b]	3.1 ± 0.2

[a] Values (IC_{50} = µM) represent mean ± SD of triplicate experiments; [b] inhibition percentage at 50 µM.

Next, the effects of compounds **4** and **5** on the kinetic profile of PTP1B-atalyzed *p*NPP hydrolysis were analyzed, as described in the methods section. When the enzyme assay was performed for the *p*NPP substrate in the presence or absence of compound **4** at different concentrations, the enzyme K_m did not change with increasing inhibitor concentration, whereas V_{max} decreased, as depicted in a Lineweaver–Burk plot in Figure 6A. Therefore, compound **4** was determined to be a noncompetitive inhibitor, suggesting that the compound may bind to an allosteric site within PTP1B or to an enzyme–substrate complex. Furthermore, the kinetic analysis revealed that the inhibition mode of compound **5** was competitive, as the Lineweaver–Burk plot showed an increase of the K_m, without changes in the V_{max} value (Figure 6B). This results indicate that compound **5** might bind to the active site of PTP1B.

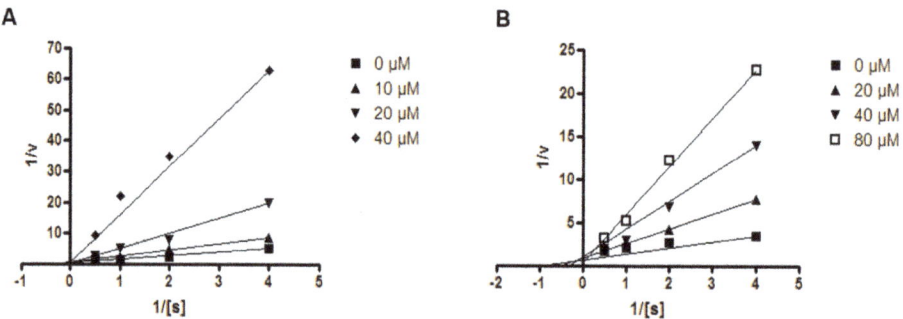

Figure 6. Lineweaver–Burk plots for compounds **4** (**A**) and **5** (**B**) representing the inhibition of PTP1B. The data represent the mean values ± SD of three experiments. The concentrations (µM) of compounds **4** and **5** are indicated.

3. Experimental

3.1. General Experimental Procedures

Optical rotations were recorded using a Jasco P-2000 digital polarimeter. NMR spectra (1D and 2D) were recorded in CD_3OD or $CDCl_3$ using a JEOL JNM ECP-400 spectrometer (400 MHz for ^1H and 100 MHz for ^{13}C) using standard JEOL pulse sequences. The chemical shifts were referenced relative to the respective residual solvent signals (CD_3OD: δ_H 3.30/δ_C 49.0 and $CDCl_3$: δ_H 7.26/δ_C 77.0). HMQC and HMBC experiments were performed using an optimized sequence for $^1J_{CH}$ = 140 Hz and $^nJ_{CH}$ = 8 Hz, respectively. HRESIMS data were obtained using an ESI Q-TOF MS/MS system (AB SCIEX Triple). HPLC separations were performed on a prep-C_{18} column (21.2 × 150 mm; 5 µm particle size) at a flow rate of 5 mL/min. UV detection at 210 nm and 254 nm was utilized. TLC analysis was performed on Kieselgel 60 F_{254} or RP-18 F_{254s} plates. Flash Column chromatography was conducted using YMC octadecyl-functionalized silica gel (C_{18}, 75 µm).

3.2. Fungal Material and Fermentation

P. glabrum SF-7123 was isolated from sediments that were collected using a dredge at the Ross Sea (77°34.397′ N, 166°10.865′ W) on 10 January 2015. One gram of the sample was mixed with sterile seawater (10 mL), and a portion (0.1 mL) of the sample was processed according to the spread plate method in potato dextrose agar (PDA) medium containing sterile seawater. The plate was incubated at 25 °C for 14 days. The isolates were cultured several times to obtain a final pure culture, and selected cultures were preserved at −70 °C. The identification of the fungal strain SF-7123 was conducted by the analysis of the 28S ribosomal RNA (rRNA) gene sequence. A GenBank search with the 28S rRNA gene of SF-7123 (GenBank accession number KY563089) indicated *P. glabrum* (JN938946), *Penicillium spinulosum* (HM469405), and *Penicillium multicolor* (HM469407) as the closest matches, showing sequence identities of 100%, 99.64%, and 97.13%, respectively. Therefore, the marine-derived fungal strain SF-7123 was characterized as *P. glabrum*.

3.3. Extraction and Isolation of Compounds **1–5**

The fungal strain SF-7123 was cultured in 10 Fernbach flasks. Each flask contained 300 mL of PDA medium with 3% NaCl (w/v). The flasks were individually inoculated with 2 mL of seed cultures of the fungal strain and incubated at 25 °C for 14 days. The fermented culture media were combined and extracted with EtOAc (4 L). The combined EtOAc extracts were then filtered through filter paper and evaporated to dryness, resulting in a crude extract of SF7123 (1.0 g). The crude extract was fractionated by reversed-phase (RP) C_{18} flash column chromatography (4.5 × 30 cm), eluting with a stepwise gradient of 20%, 30%, 40%, 50%, 60%, 80%, and 100% (v/v) MeOH in H_2O (400 mL each) to provide seven subfractions, SF7123-1 to SF7123-8. Fraction SF7123-4 was subjected to column chromatography (3 × 35 cm) using Sephadex LH-20 as the stationary phase and a 3/1 (v/v) mixture of MeOH in water as the mobile phase to provide metabolite **4** (2.5 mg) and two sub-fractions named SF7123-4-1 and SF7123-4-2. Subfraction SF7123-4-2 was then chromatographed using an RP C_{18} column (1.2 × 30 cm) and eluted with MeOH in water [2/3 (v/v)] to create three subfractions. Among these subfractions, subfraction SF7123-4-2-1 was further separated on a C_{18} prep HPLC (27%–43% CH_3CN in H_2O (0.1% HCOOH) over 16 min) to provide metabolite **2** (6.5 mg, t_R = 15 min). Similarly, subfraction SF7123-4-2-2 was purified by using C_{18} prep HPLC (35%–50% CH_3CN in H_2O (0.1% HCOOH) over 16 min) to afford metabolite **1** (4.3 mg, t_R = 15.5 min). Fraction SF7123-5 was subjected to column chromatography using Sephadex LH-20 (2.0 × 30 cm). The column was subsequently eluted with a mixture of MeOH in H_2O [3/1 (v/v)] to separate the fraction into three subfractions, i.e., SF7123-5-1 to SF7123-5-3. The first subfraction, SF7123-5-1, was subjected to C_{18} prep HPLC (48%–70% CH_3CN in water (0.1% HCOOH) over 18 min) to afford compound **5** (6 mg, t_R = 17.0 min). Compound **3** (2 mg, t_R = 23.0 min) was isolated from the second subfraction, SF7123-5-2, by RP C_{18} prep HPLC (35%–65% CH_3CN in H_2O (0.1% HCOOH) over 25 min).

Compound 9-O-methylneuchromenin (**1**): Yellow powder; $[\alpha]_D$ −344 (c = 0.72, MeOH); ^{1}H and ^{13}C NMR data, see Table 1; HRESIMS m/z: 263.0911 [M + H]$^+$ (calcd. for $C_{14}H_{15}O_5$, 263.0919).

3.4. Cell Culture and Viability Assay

RAW264.7 and BV2 cells were maintained at 5 × 10^5 cells/mL in Dulbecco's modified Eagle's medium (DMEM) containing 10% fetal bovine serum (FBS), penicillin G (100 U/mL), streptomycin (100 mg/L), and L-glutamine (2 mM) and incubated at 37 °C in a humidified atmosphere containing 5% CO_2. DMEM, FBS, and other tissue culture reagents were purchased from Gibco BRL Co. Cell viability was evaluated by the MTT assay as described in our previous report [30].

3.5. Nitrite Determination

To determine the nitrite concentration in the medium as an indicator of NO production, the Griess reaction was carried out as described in our previous report [30].

3.6. Preparation of Cytosolic and Nuclear Fractions

An Affymetrix Nuclear Extraction kit (Affymetrix Inc., Santa Clara, CA, USA) was used to extract the cytosolic and nuclear fractions of the cells. The lysis of each fraction was conducted according to the manufacturer's instructions. The details regarding the preparation of the cytosolic and nuclear fractions have been described previously [30].

3.7. Western Blot Analysis

Western blot analysis was carried out according to our previous report [30]. Briefly, cells were harvested by centrifugation at 200 g for 3 min, followed by a washing step with RIPA lysis buffer (25 mM Tris-HCl buffer (pH 7.6), 150 mM NaCl, 1% NP-40, 1% sodium deoxycholate, and 0.1% SDS). Primary antibodies (COX-2: sc-1745; iNOS: sc-650; IκB-α: sc-371; p-IκB-α: sc-8404; p50: sc-7178; and p65: sc-8008) were purchased from Santa Cruz Biotechnology, and secondary antibodies (mouse: ap124p; goat: ap106p; and rabbit: ap132p) were purchased from Millipore.

3.8. DNA-Binding Activity of NF-κB

The DNA-binding activity of NF-κB in the nuclear extracts was measured using the TransAM® kit (Active Motif, Carlsbad, CA, USA); three independent assays for each sample were conducted according to the manufacturer's instructions.

3.9. PGE_2 Assay

The level of PGE_2 present in each sample was determined using a commercially available kit from R&D Systems (Minneapolis, MN, USA); the details of this assay were described previously [30]. Three independent assays were performed according to the manufacturer's instructions.

3.10. Quantitative Real-Time Reverse-Transcription PCR (qRT-PCR)

Triplicate quantitative reverse-transcription polymerase chain reaction analysis was conducted using the following primers: 5'-AAT TGG TCA TAG CCC GCA CT-3' and 5'-AAG CAA TGT GCT GGT GCT TC-3, forward and reverse primers for IL-1β, 5'-CCA GAC CCT CAC ACT CAC AA-3' and 5'-ACA AGG TAC AAC CCA TCG GC-3', forward and reverse primers for TNF-α, 5'-ACT TCA CAA GTC GGA GGC TT-3' and 5'-TGC AAG TGC ATC ATC GTT GT-3', forward and reverse primers for IL-6, 5'-AGT GAC ATG TGG AAT GGC GT-3' and 5'-CAG TTC AAT GGG CAG GGT CT-3, forward and reverse primers for IL-12, and 5'-ACT TTG GTA TCG TGG AAG GAC T-3' and 5'-GTA GAG GCA GGG ATG ATG TTC T-3', forward and reverse primers for GADPH. The optimum conditions for PCR amplification of the cDNAs were according to the manufacturer's instructions; the details of this assay have been previously reported [30].

3.11. PTP1B Assay

PTP1B (human, recombinant) used in the current study was purchased from BIOMOL Research Laboratories, Inc. PTP1B enzyme activity was determined using 2 mM of *p*NPP as a substrate in 50 mM citrate buffer solution (pH 6.0, 0.1 M NaCl, 1 mM EDTA, and 1 mM dithiothreitol). The reaction mixture was incubated at 30 °C for 30 min, and the reaction was terminated by the addition of 1 N NaOH. The amount of *p*-nitrophenol produced by the enzyme was estimated by measuring the increase in absorbance at 405 nm. The nonenzymatic hydrolysis of 2 mM *p*NPP was corrected by measuring the increase in absorbance at 405 nm in the absence of PTP1B [31]. The kinetic analysis involved the following: the assays were performed using a reaction mixture that contained different concentrations of *p*NPP (0.25 mM, 0.5 mM, 1.0 mM, and 2.0 mM) as a PTP1B substrate in the absence or presence of compounds **4** and **5**. The Michaelis–Menten constant (K_m) and maximum velocity (V_{max}) of PTP1B were determined by the Lineweaver–Burk plot using the GraphPad Prism® 4 program (GraphPad Software Inc., San Diego, CA, USA).

3.12. Statistical Analysis

Each experiment was performed at least three times independently, and the resulting data are presented as the mean ± standard deviation. The comparison of three or more groups utilized one-way analysis of variance (ANOVA), followed by Tukey's multiple comparison tests. Statistical analysis was performed using GraphPad Prism software, version 3.03 (GraphPad Software Inc, GraphPad Software Inc., San Diego, CA, USA).

4. Conclusions

In summary, our chemical investigation of the marine-derived fungal isolate *P. glabrum* SF-7123 resulted in the isolation and identification of five secondary metabolites, including one new fungal metabolite named 9-*O*-methylneuchromenin (**1**). Although several biological activities of some known metabolites described in this study have already been reported, their anti-inflammatory, anti-neuroinflammatory, and PTP1B inhibitory effects had not yet been investigated. Our results demonstrated that compounds **2**, **4**, and **5** inhibited LPS-induced overproduction of NO and PGE_2 in BV2 microglial and RAW264.7 macrophage cells. Among these compounds, compound **2** was identified as the most active compound. Furthermore, compound **2** attenuated the mRNA expression of pro-inflammatory cytokines and the protein expression of iNOS and COX-2 in BV2 and RAW264.7 cells. Furthermore, the inhibitory effects of **2** were associated with the inactivation of NF-κB and p38 MAPK pathways. It is noteworthy that a minor modification of the dihydropyranobenzopyranone skeleton in compounds **1** and **2** produced a significant variation in the anti-inflammatory effect in the cellular models considered. This result suggests that this class of compound should be the subject of further investigation, particularly regarding structure and activity relationship. In addition, compounds **4** and **5**, which, respectively, are dihydropyranochromenone- and benzoylpyronone-type metabolites, have properties that suggest their pharmacologically evaluation for the treatment of diseases related to the regulation of PTP1B activity. According to the Michaelis –Menten kinetic model, compound **4** was identified as a noncompetitive inhibitor of the PTP1B enzyme, and compound **5** appeared to be a competitive inhibitor of this enzyme. Thus, this study demonstrates the potential value of marine-derived fungal isolates as a bioresource for bioactive compounds. The metabolites identified in this study should be further evaluated for their putative pharmacological properties.

Supplementary Materials: The following are available online at http://www.mdpi.com/1660-3397/18/5/247/s1, Figures S1–S9: 1D NMR, 2D NMR, and HRESIMS spectra of the new compound **1**, and ^{1}H NMR spectra of compounds **2**–**5** are supplied.

Author Contributions: T.M.H. contributed to the isolation of the compounds and wrote the manuscript; D.-C.K. performed the experiments related to the biological evaluation of the compounds and wrote the manuscript; J.H.S. isolated and identified the fungal strains; J.H.Y. organized this work, collected and provided the Antarctic sample, and wrote the manuscript; H.O. organized this work, contributed to the isolation and structure determination of the compounds, and wrote the manuscript. All authors have read and agreed to the published version of the manuscript.

Funding: This work was supported by a grant from the Korea Polar Research Institute (PE20010).

Conflicts of Interest: The authors declare that they have no conflicts of interest.

References

1. Ebada, S.S.; Proksch, P. *Marine-Derived Fungal Metabolites*; Kim, S.K., Ed.; Springer: Berlin/Heidelberg, Germany, 2015; pp. 759–788.
2. Jin, L.; Quan, C.; Hou, X.; Fan, S. Potential Pharmacological Resources: Natural Bioactive Compounds from Marine-Derived Fungi. *Mar. Drugs* **2016**, *14*, 76. [CrossRef] [PubMed]
3. Rateb, M.E.; Ebel, R. Secondary metabolites of fungi from marine habitats. *Nat. Prod. Rep.* **2011**, *28*, 290–344. [CrossRef] [PubMed]
4. Block, M.L.; Zecca, L.; Hong, J.S. Microglia-mediated neurotoxicity: Uncovering the molecular mechanisms. *Nat. Rev. Neurosci.* **2007**, *8*, 57–69. [CrossRef] [PubMed]

5. Sugama, S. Stress-induced microglial activation may facilitate the progression of neurodegenerative disorders. *Med. Hypotheses* **2009**, *73*, 1031–1034. [CrossRef] [PubMed]
6. Lappas, M.; Permezel, M.; Georgiou, H.M.; Rice, G.E. Nuclear factor kappa B regulation of proinflammatory cytokines in human gestational tissues in vitro. *Biol. Reprod.* **2002**, *67*, 668–673. [CrossRef] [PubMed]
7. Amor, S.; Puentes, F.; Baker, D.; van der Valk, P. Inflammation in neurodegenerative diseases. *Immunology* **2010**, *129*, 154–169. [CrossRef]
8. Lue, L.F.; Kuo, Y.M.; Beach, T.; Walker, D.G. Microglia activation and anti-inflammatory regulation in Alzheimer's disease. *Mol. Neurobiol.* **2010**, *41*, 115–128. [CrossRef]
9. Long-Smith, C.M.; Sullivan, A.M.; Nolan, Y.M. The influence of microglia on the pathogenesis of Parkinson's disease. *Prog. Neurobiol.* **2009**, *89*, 277–287. [CrossRef]
10. Tsunekawa, T.; Banno, R.; Mizoguchi, A.; Sugiyama, M.; Tominaga, T.; Onoue, T.; Hagiwara, D.; Ito, Y.; Iwama, S.; Goto, M.; et al. Deficiency of PTP1B Attenuates Hypothalamic Inflammation via Activation of the JAK2-STAT3 Pathway in Microglia. *EBioMedicine* **2017**, *16*, 172–183. [CrossRef]
11. Erdnikovs, S.; Abdala-Valencia, H.; Cook-Mills, J.M. ndothelial cell PTP1B regulates leukocyte recruitment during allergic inflammation. *Am. J. Physiol. Lung Cell Mol. Physiol.* **2013**, *304*, 240–249. [CrossRef]
12. Song, G.J.; Jung, M.; Kim, J.H.; Park, H.; Rahman, M.H.; Zhang, S.; Zhang, Z.Y.; Park, D.H.; Kook, H.; Lee, I.K.; et al. A novel role for protein tyrosine phosphatase 1B as a positive regulator of neuroinflammation. *J. Neuroinflamm.* **2016**, *13*, 86. [CrossRef] [PubMed]
13. Tanada, Y.; Mori, K. Synthesis and absolute configuration of (-)-neuchromenin, a neurotrophic metabolite of *Eupenicillin javanicum* var. *meloforme*, and its enantiomer. *Eur. J. Org. Chem.* **2001**, *2001*, 1963–1966. [CrossRef]
14. Hayakawa, Y.; Yamamoto, H.; Tsuge, N.; Seto, H. Structure of a new microbial metabolite, neuchromenin. *Tetrahedron Lett.* **1996**, *37*, 6363–6364. [CrossRef]
15. Tanada, Y.; Mori, K. Synthesis and absolute configuration of Nocardione A and B, furano-o-naphthoquinone-type metabolites of nocardia sp with antifungal, cytotoxic, and enzyme inhibitory activities. *Eur. J. Org. Chem.* **2001**, *2001*, 4313–4319. [CrossRef]
16. Liao, W.Y.; Shen, C.N.; Lin, L.H.; Yang, Y.L.; Han, H.Y.; Chen, J.W.; Kuo, S.C.; Wu, S.H.; Liaw, C.C. Asperjinone, a nor-neolignan, and terrein, a suppressor of ABCG2-expressing breast cancer cells, from thermophilic Aspergillus terreus. *J. Nat. Prod.* **2012**, *75*, 630–635. [CrossRef]
17. Ohashi, H.; Akiyama, H.; Nishikori, K.; Mochizuki, J. Asterric acid, a new endothelin binding inhibitor. *J. Antibiot.* **1992**, *45*, 1684–1685. [CrossRef]
18. Yuan, C.; Wang, H.Y.; Wu, C.S.; Jiao, Y.; Li, M.; Wang, Y.Y.; Wang, S.Q.; Zhao, Z.T.; Lou, H.X. Austdiol, fulvic acid and citromycetin derivatives from an endolichenic fungus, *Myxotrichum* sp. *Phytochem. Lett.* **2013**, *6*, 662–666. [CrossRef]
19. Sassa, T.; Nukina, M.; Suzuki, Y. Deoxyfunicone, a New γ-Pyrone Metabolite from a Resorcylide-producing Fungus (*Penicillium* sp). *Agric. Biol. Chem.* **1991**, *55*, 2415–2416.
20. Singh, S.B.; Jayasuriya, H.; Dewey, R.; Polishook, J.D.; Dombrowski, A.W.; Zink, D.L.; Guan, Z.; Collado, J.; Platas, G.; Pelaez, F.; et al. Isolation, structure, and HIV-1-integrase inhibitory activity of structurally diverse fungal metabolites. *J. Ind. Microbiol. Biotechnol.* **2003**, *30*, 721–731.
21. Zhang, H.; Shan, Y.; Wu, Y.; Xu, C.; Yu, X.; Zhao, J.; Yan, J.; Shang, W. Berberine suppresses LPS-induced inflammation through modulating Sirt1/NF-κB signaling pathway in RAW264.7 cells. *Int. Immunopharmacol.* **2017**, *52*, 93–100. [CrossRef]
22. Jung, E.H.; Hwang, J.S.; Kwon, M.Y.; Kim, K.H.; Cho, H.; Lyoo, I.K.; Shin, S.; Park, J.H.; Han, I.O. A tryptamine-paeonol hybridization compound inhibits LPS-mediated inflammation in BV2 cells. *Neurochem. Int.* **2016**, *100*, 35–43. [CrossRef]
23. Siebenlist, U.; Franzoso, G.; Brown, K. Structure, regulation and function of NF-kappa B. *Annu. Rev. Cell Biol.* **1994**, *10*, 405–455. [CrossRef]
24. Karin, M.; Ben-Neriah, Y. Phosphorylation meets ubiquitination: The control of NF-[kappa]B activity. *Annu. Rev. Immunol.* **2000**, *18*, 621–663. [CrossRef]
25. Ghosh, S.; May, M.J.; Kopp, E.B. NF-kappa B and Rel proteins: Evolutionarily conserved mediators of immune responses. *Annu. Rev. Immunol.* **1998**, *16*, 225–260. [CrossRef]
26. Liu, Y.; Shepherd, E.G.; Nelin, L.D. MAPK phosphatases–regulating the immune response. *Nat. Rev. Immunol.* **2007**, *7*, 202–212. [CrossRef]

27. Dong, C.; Davis, R.J.; Flavell, R.A. MAP kinases in the immune response. *Annu. Rev. Immunol.* **2002**, *20*, 55–72. [CrossRef]
28. Na, M.; Tang, S.; He, L.; Oh, H.; Kim, B.S.; Oh, W.K.; Kim, B.Y.; Ahn, J.S. Inhibition of protein tyrosine phosphatase 1B by ursane-type triterpenes isolated from Symplocos paniculata. *Planta Med.* **2006**, *72*, 261–263. [CrossRef]
29. Zhang, W.; Hong, D.; Zhou, Y.; Zhang, Y.; Shen, Q.; Li, J.; Hu, L.; Li, J. Ursolic acid and its derivative inhibit protein tyrosine phosphatase 1B, enhancing insulin receptor phosphorylation and stimulating glucose uptake. *Biochem. Biophys. Acta* **2006**, *1760*, 1505–1512. [CrossRef] [PubMed]
30. Cho, K.H.; Kim, D.C.; Yoon, C.S.; Ko, W.M.; Lee, S.J.; Sohn, J.H.; Jang, J.H.; Ahn, J.S.; Kim, Y.C.; Oh, H. Anti-neuroinflammatory effects of citreohybridonol involving TLR4-MyD88-mediated inhibition of NF-κB and MAPK signaling pathways in lipopolysaccharide-stimulated BV2 cells. *Neurochem. Int.* **2016**, *95*, 55–62. [CrossRef] [PubMed]
31. Hamaguchi, T.; Sudo, T.; Osada, H. RK-682, a potent inhibitor of tyrosine phosphatase, arrested the mammalian cell cycle progression at G1phase. *FEBS Lett.* **1995**, *372*, 54–58. [CrossRef]

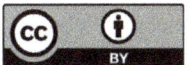

© 2020 by the authors. Licensee MDPI, Basel, Switzerland. This article is an open access article distributed under the terms and conditions of the Creative Commons Attribution (CC BY) license (http://creativecommons.org/licenses/by/4.0/).

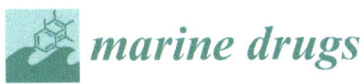

Article

Proteoglycan from *Bacillus* sp. BS11 Inhibits the Inflammatory Response by Suppressing the MAPK and NF-κB Pathways in Lipopolysaccharide-Induced RAW264.7 Macrophages

Qingchi Wang [1,2,3,4], Weixiang Liu [1,2,3,4], Yang Yue [1,2,3,4], Chaomin Sun [1,2,3,4] and Quanbin Zhang [1,2,3,4,*]

1. CAS Key Laboratory of Experimental Marine Biology, Institute of Oceanology, Chinese Academy of Sciences, Qingdao 266071, China; wangqingchi@qdio.ac.cn (Q.W.); liuweixiang@qdio.ac.cn (W.L.); yueyang@qdio.ac.cn (Y.Y.); sunchaomin@qdio.ac.cn (C.S.)
2. Laboratory for Marine Biology and Biotechnology, Qingdao National Laboratory for Marine Science and Technology, Qingdao 266071, China
3. Department of Earth Science, University of Chinese Academy of Sciences, Beijing 100049, China
4. Center for Ocean Mega-Science, Chinese Academy of Sciences, Qingdao 266071, China
* Correspondence: qbzhang@qdio.ac.cn; Tel./Fax: +86-532-8289-8708

Received: 12 October 2020; Accepted: 20 November 2020; Published: 24 November 2020

Abstract: Inflammation is involved in the pathogenesis of many debilitating diseases. Proteoglycan isolated from marine *Bacillus* sp. BS11 (EPS11) was shown to have anticancer activity, but its anti-inflammatory potential remains elusive. In the present study, the anti-inflammatory effects and mechanism of EPS11 were evaluated using a lipopolysaccharide (LPS)-induced RAW264.7 macrophage model. Biochemical characterization showed that the total sugar content and protein content of EPS11 were 49.5% and 30.2% respectively. EPS11 was composed of mannose, glucosamine, galactosamine, glucose, galactose, rhamnose, and glucuronic acid. Its molecular weight was determined to be 3.06×10^5 Da. The protein determination of EPS11 was also performed. EPS11 displayed a strong anti-inflammatory effect on LPS-stimulated RAW264.7 macrophages in vitro, which significantly suppressed inflammatory cytokines and mediators (such as NO, TNF-α, IL-6 and IL-1β, and COX-2). Western blot analysis indicated that EPS11 could downregulate the expression of many key proteins in mitogen-activated protein kinases (MAPKs) and transcription factor nuclear factor-κB (NF-κB) signaling pathways. In particular, EPS11 almost completely inhibited the expression of NF-κB P65, which indicated that EPS11 acted primarily on the NF-κB pathways. These findings offer new insights into the molecular mechanism underlying the anti-inflammatory effect of EPS11.

Keywords: *Bacillus* sp.; proteoglycan; anti-inflammation; macrophages

1. Introduction

The immune system has multiple functions, including recognition, elimination, and regulation, which are beneficial for organisms. However, the dysregulation of the immune system may cause many pathological immune responses, such as inflammation, allergy, and asthma [1]. Inflammation has been especially linked with the pathogenesis of many diseases, such as arthritis, cancer, neurodegenerative disease, cardiovascular disease, and multiple sclerosis [2–7]. Therefore, a number of chemically synthesized compounds were used as immunomodulators to regulate the immune system [8,9]. Due to some adverse events, such as toxic effects on the liver, lungs, kidneys, and gastrointestinal tract, their clinical applications are restricted [10]. In recent years, much attention has been paid to natural polysaccharides due to their nontoxic properties and immunomodulatory activities [11–13].

Macrophages act as the first line of defense in the immune system, and display extensive biological functions such as phagocytosis, the destruction of pathogens, antigen presentation, and cytokine production [14]. Many external stimuli, such as lipopolysaccharides (LPS), carbohydrates, and some cytokines can interact with the pattern-recognition receptors of macrophages. Then, a series of intracellular responses are activated, and several related signaling pathways, including transcription factors nuclear factor-κB (NF-κB) and mitogen-activated protein kinases (MAPKs) may be involved in signal transmission [15,16]. During inflammation, macrophages execute their function of immune response by producing various inflammatory cytokines and mediators [17,18], such as tumor necrosis factor (TNF-α), transforming growth factor-β (TGF-β), interleukin-1 (IL-1), interleukin-6 (IL-6), prostaglandin E2 (PGE2), and nitric oxide (NO) [19,20]. In turn, these inflammatory mediators promote the development of inflammation. Thus, compounds that can reduce inflammatory mediators may be developed into therapeutic agents for inflammatory diseases.

Proteoglycan (EPS11) was sourced from marine *Bacillus* sp. BS11, which was reported to inhibit cancer-cell growth via blocking cell adhesion in previous studies [21,22]. However, the inflammatory effects and mechanism of EPS11 were not investigated. In this study, EPS11 was prepared, and its structural features were determined by chemical analysis. The in vitro immunomodulatory effect of EPS11 was investigated by determining the inhibition of inflammatory mediators produced by LPS-activated RAW 264.7 macrophages. The mechanisms of EPS11 acting on MAPKs and NF-κB signaling pathways were also explored.

2. Results

2.1. Extraction and Purification of EPS11

The extraction and purification of EPS11 was carried out as described in Section 4.2. The polysaccharide fraction and protein fraction were detected by sulfuric acid–phenol method and UV detector, respectively (Figure 1). The results showed that the eluted peak was relatively high and symmetrical when NaCl concentration was 250 mmol/L (Figure 1A,C). Then, this peak was collected, concentrated, and purified by HiLoad^{TM} 16/600 Superdex^{TM} 200 gel-column chromatography (Figure 1B,D). The highest peak in gel chromatography was collected to concentrate, dialyze, and lyophilize, and it was labeled as EPS11.

2.2. Physicochemical-Property Analysis of EPS11

Table 1 shows that total sugar content is 49.5%, which was determined using Man as the standard. The protein content was 30.2% and the moisture content was 5.6%. The results showed that EPS11 is a proteoglycan. The results of amino acid analysis showed that EPS11 contained 20 kinds of amino acids, and the total amino acid content was 30.5%, which was consistent with the results of protein content (Table 2).

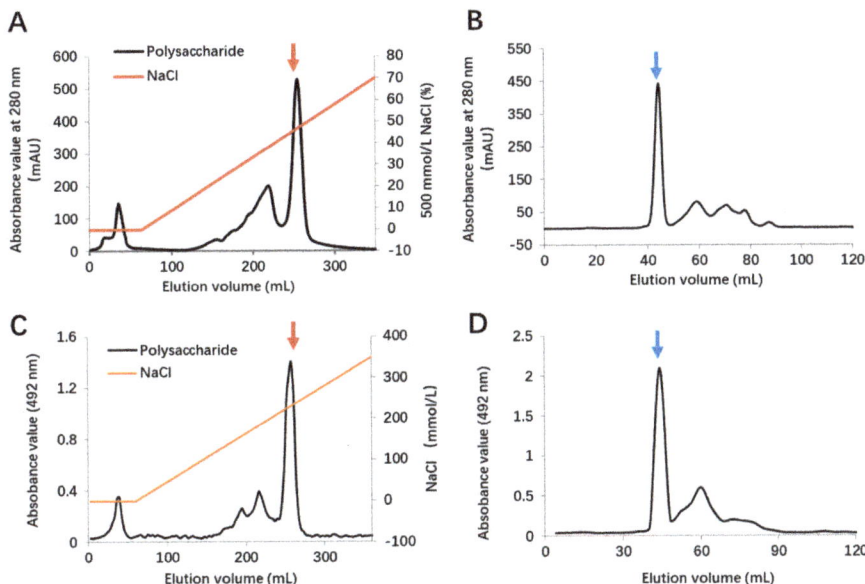

Figure 1. Purification of marine *Bacillus* sp. BS11 (EPS11). (**A**) Elution spectra of diethylaminoethyl cellulose (DEAE) Fast Flow ion-exchange column chromatography of protein. (**B**) Elution spectra of HiLoad™ 16/600 Superdex™ 200 gel-column chromatography of first purified fraction (red arrow in (**A**)). (**C**) Elution spectra of diethylaminoethyl cellulose (DEAE) Fast Flow ion-exchange column chromatography of crude polysaccharide. (**D**) Elution spectra of HiLoad™ 16/600 Superdex™ 200 gel-column chromatography of first purified fraction (red arrow in (**C**)). Final purified fraction (blue arrow) was collected, dialyzed, and lyophilized.

Table 1. Chemical analysis of EPS11.

EPS11	
Total sugar content	49.5%
Protein content	30.2%
Moisture content	5.6%
Average molecular weight (Da)	3.06×10^5
Monosaccharide composition (molar ratio)	
Mannose (Man)	13.08
Glucosamine (GlcN)	7.84
Rhamnose (Rha)	1.00
Glucuronic acid (GlcA)	1.03
Galactosamine (GalN)	8.23
Glucose (Glc)	4.73
Galactose (Gal)	7.03

The chromatograms of monosaccharide standards and EPS11-sourced hydrolysate are presented in Figure 2A,B. EPS11 was composed of mannose (Man), glucosamine (GlcN), galactosamine (GalN), glucose (Glc), galactose (Gal), rhamnose (Rha), and glucuronic acid (GlcA) with detected molar ratio as 13.08:7.84:8.23:4.73:7.03:1.00:1.03 (Table 1). The results showed that Man was the dominant monosaccharide in EPS11, and GlcN, GalN, Glc, and Gal were also present in EPS11 with relatively high abundance. As shown in Figure 2C, the peak of EPS11 at 13.762 min was single and symmetrical, and average molecular weight was determined for 3.06×10^5 Da (Table 1).

Table 2. Amino acid composition of EPS11.

No.	Name	Retention Time (min)	Peak Area	Content (% of Total Sample)
1	Aspartic acid (Asp)	9.11	18,383.87	3.76
2	Threonine (Thr)	11.17	5331.41	0.90
3	Serine (Ser)	12.05	23,249.59	3.70
4	Glutamic acid (Glu)	13.81	35,477.82	8.46
5	Glycine (Gly)	19.95	18,134.89	2.05
6	Alanine (Ala)	21.30	12,356.06	1.65
7	Cysteic acid (Cys)	22.73	406.54	0.25
8	Valine (Val)	23.94	6759.21	1.17
9	Methionine (Met)	26.09	785.08	0.18
10	Isoleucine (Ile)	28.68	6223.54	1.23
11	Leucine (Leu)	29.88	4052.47	0.80
12	Tyrosine (Tyr)	32.22	1479.20	0.41
13	Phenylalanine (Phe)	33.38	1476.18	0.37
14	Histidine (His)	36.59	11,132.71	2.55
15	Lysine (Lys)	29.68	4326.45	0.93
16	Arginine (Arg)	44.22	1960.02	0.58
17	Proline (Pro)	15.33	1684.57	1.55
	Total		153,219.60	30.52

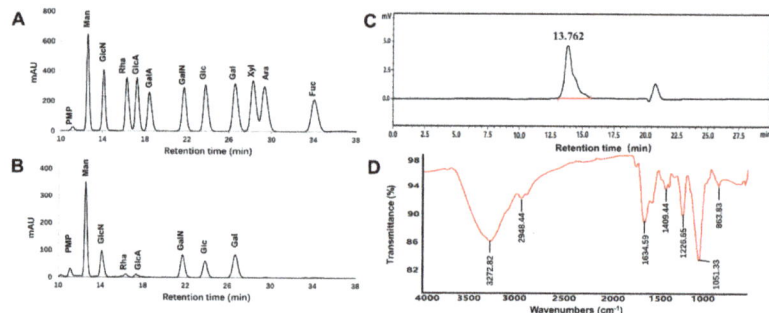

Figure 2. Physicochemical properties of EPS11. (**A**) Chromatography of monosaccharides with mixed standards including eleven sugars (Man, GlcN, Rha, GlcA, GalA, GalN, Glc, Gal, Xyl, Ara, Fuc). (**B**) Chromatography of EPS11 for monosaccharide-composition analysis. (**C**) Chromatography of EPS11 for molecular-weight determination. (**D**) FT–IR spectrum of EPS11.

The FT–IR spectrum of EPS11 presented in Figure 2D showed the characteristic absorption. The broad intense peak at 3272 cm^{-1} and a weak peak around 2948 cm^{-1} represented the stretching vibration of O–H or N–H bonds and C–H bonds in the sugar ring, respectively. Strong peaks at 1634 and 1540 cm^{-1} were associated with the stretching vibration of C=O or formation vibration of N–H. This indicated that aminosaccharides or protein were present. The narrow intense peak at 1051 cm^{-1} represented the stretching vibration of C–O–C or C–O–H. Peaks at 1225 and 836 cm^{-1} implied that the sulfate group might have been present.

2.3. Protein Profiling of EPS11 by LC-MS/MS

To investigate the composition of protein contained in EPS11, LC-MS/MS analysis was carried out. The results showed that a total of 41 peptides were obtained by enzymatic hydrolysis from EPS11. The sequences of the peptides are shown as follow: AFSEDGGTDIDLLEAGEWIIAPK; AFSEDGGTDIDLLEAGEWIIAPKDAEGNPHPEK; AGENVGVLLR; AIDKPFLLPIEDVFSISGR; AIQEPNCLEATIAPSGHK; ALVTGGLFR; APDVVNNSWGGGPGLDEWYR; APDVVNNSWGGGPGLDEWYRPMVQNWR; APEEEGNYMIR; DAEGNPHPEK; DAEGNPHPEKA PDVVNNSWGGGPGLDEWYR; DAEGNPHPEKAPDVVNNSWGGGPGLDEWYRPMVQNWR; DAE

GNPHPELAPDVVNNSWGGGPGLDEWYRPMVQNWR; DSFGNETRK; DSYVGDEAQSK; EITAL APATMK; FWNTEWPNPGGTNFK; GDVHDENLAWVK; GYRPQFYFR;HQGVMVGMGQK; HTP FFK;HYAHVDCPGHADYVK; IWHHTFYNELR; KTAEGLLNINTK; LCYVALDFEQEMATAASSSSLEK; MSLAEGQER; PDVSAPGVNIR; PMVQNWR; QEYDESGPSIVHR; QLELLEKMRDMNASLSK; SYELPDGQVITIGNER; TTLTAAITTVLAK; VAPEEHPVLLTEAPLNPK; VEIHDASGPDGAPGK; VGAPEVWDMGIDGAGTVIANIDTGVQWDHPALMEQYR; VKDSFGNETR; VKDSFGNETRK; VLT GGVDANALQRPK; YHEEIPLR; YTLAGTEVSALLGR. After mass spectrometry data retrieval and screening, the potential proteins in EPS11 showed some homology with the identified eight proteins, which are shown in the Table 3. The two proteins with the highest matching scores were Bacillopeptidase F and Actin. Bacillopeptidase F is a serine endopeptidase, which was first isolated from Bacillus subtilis. Actin is commonly found in eukaryotic cells and is encoded by highly conserved genes.

Table 3. Protein analysis of EPS11.

No.	Majority Protein IDs	Protein Names	Sequence Coverage [%]	Mol. Weight [kDa]	Score
1	A0A2A9CJM4	Bacillopeptidase F	14.1	155.94	323.31
2	A0A6I2ACB9	Actin, cytoplasmic 2	30.3	41.71	119.44
3	A0A2L0R4Y2	Elongation factor Tu (Fragment)	21.4	43.05	44.24
4	A0A5A9E4B1	S8 family serine peptidase	2.8	147.43	14.79
5	A0A2S9WBY3; A0A328LLM6	F0F1 ATP synthase subunit beta (Fragment)	10.7	14.17	12.54
6	A0A2A9CFX8	Spore coat protein E	14.1	21.01	12.15
7	A0A328M8Z8	Transcription termination factor Rho	2.5	66.63	8.49
8	A0A4U1CWZ7	Unnamed (Gene names: FA727_21720)	8.9	22.85	−2.00

2.4. Effects of EPS11 on RAW264.7 Macrophage Viability

To evaluate the effect of EPS11 on the viability of RAW264.7 macrophages, the macrophages were treated with EPS11 (6.25–200 µg/mL) or LPS (1.0 µg/mL) for 24 h. The control group was designated as 100% cell viability. The results showed that EPS11 had no cytotoxicity with RAW264.7 macrophages at the tested concentrations (6.25–200 µg/mL; Figure 3A). Figure 3B displays that RAW264.7 macrophages were coincubated with EPS11 and LPS, and cell viability exceeded 75% in all groups, indicating that EPS11 was nontoxic to RAW264.7 macrophages. Therefore, these concentrations (6.25–200 µg/mL) were used for the following experiments.

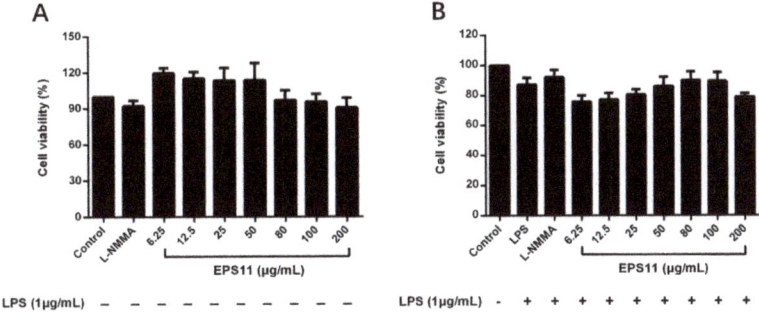

Figure 3. Effect of EPS11 on RAW 264.7 macrophage viability. (A) Macrophages cultured by EPS11 (6.25, 12.5, 25, 50, 80, 100, and 200 µg/mL) alone for 24 h. (B) Macrophages cotreated by EPS11 (6.25, 12.5, 25, 50, 80, 100, and 200 µg/mL) and lipopolysaccharides (LPS; 1 µg/mL) for 24 h. Data presented as means ± SD (n = 3) from independent experiments.

2.5. Active Fraction Appraisal

To identify the active fraction, LPS-induced RAW264.7 macrophages were treated with EPS11 (200 µg/mL) which was treated by proteinase K and NaIO4, respectively. The results showed that there was no significant effect on the inhibition of NO production with EPS11 treated by proteinase K. However, the cells incubated with NaIO4-treated EPS11 increased NO production as the same as LPS group (Figure 4). The results suggested that the anti-inflammatory activity of EPS11 is due to the polysaccharide fraction.

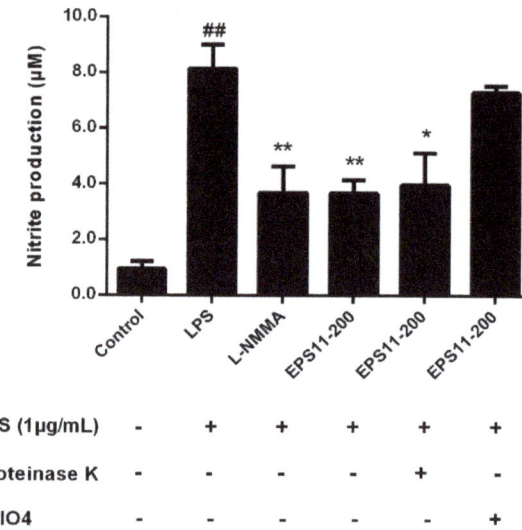

Figure 4. Identification of active fraction of EPS11. EPS11 (200 µg/mL) was. LPS-induced RAW264.7 macrophages were incubated with EPS11 that was treated with proteinase K (50 µg/mL) and NaIO4 (15 mmol/L), respectively. The levels of NO production were detected to evaluate the anti-inflammatory activity of each fraction. Data presented as mean ± SE (n = 3) from independent experiments. Significance: ## $p < 0.01$ vs. control; * $p < 0.05$, ** $p < 0.01$ vs. LPS-treated.

2.6. EPS11 Inhibits NO Production

NO, as an important indicator of inflammation, is produced and regulated by nitric oxide synthase (iNOS) [23]. As shown in Figure 5A, EPS11 inhibited the generation of NO in LPS-induced RAW264.7 macrophages in a concentration-dependent manner. In particular, macrophages treated with EPS11 (50–200 µg/mL) showed significantly lower NO production than that in the control. NO inhibitory effects of positive controls aspirin (200 µg/mL) and NG-monomethyl-L-arginine, monoacetate salt (L-NMMA) (50 µmol/L) were also observed. Figure 5B shows that EPS11 with different concentrations did not influence the generation of NO in RAW264.7 macrophages without LPS stimulation, which indicated that EPS11 may act by influencing NO production-related signaling pathways.

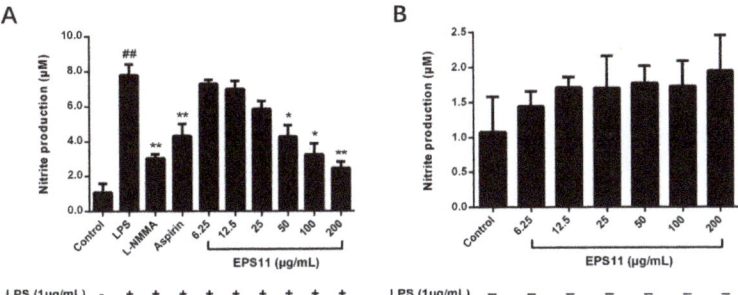

Figure 5. Effect of EPS11 on NO production in RAW264.7 macrophages. (**A**) Macrophages cotreated with EPS11 (6.25, 12.5, 25, 50, 100, and 200 µg/mL) and LPS (1.0 µg/mL) for 24 h. (**B**) Macrophages treated with EPS11 (6.25, 12.5, 25, 50, 100, and 200 µg/mL) alone for 24 h. Data presented as mean ± SE (n = 3) from independent experiments. Significance: ## $p < 0.01$ vs. control; * $p < 0.05$, ** $p < 0.01$ vs. LPS-treated.

2.7. EPS11 Decreases Expression of COX-2, TNF-α, IL-1β, and IL-6

The inhibitory effects of EPS11 on COX-2, TNF-α, IL-1β, and IL-6 levels were further investigated. Figure 6 shows that LPS (1.0 µg/mL) significantly increased the expression of COX-2 and cytokines in macrophages. However, the production of TNF-α in supernatants of the EPS11-treated macrophages was significantly decreased in a concentration-dependent manner (Figure 6A). Similarly, the inhibitory effects of EPS11 on IL-1β, IL-6, and COX-2 in LPS-induced RAW264.7 macrophages were also observed (Figure 6B–D). Therefore, these observations suggested that EPS11 may inhibit the protein expression of COX-2, TNF-α, IL-1β, and IL-6.

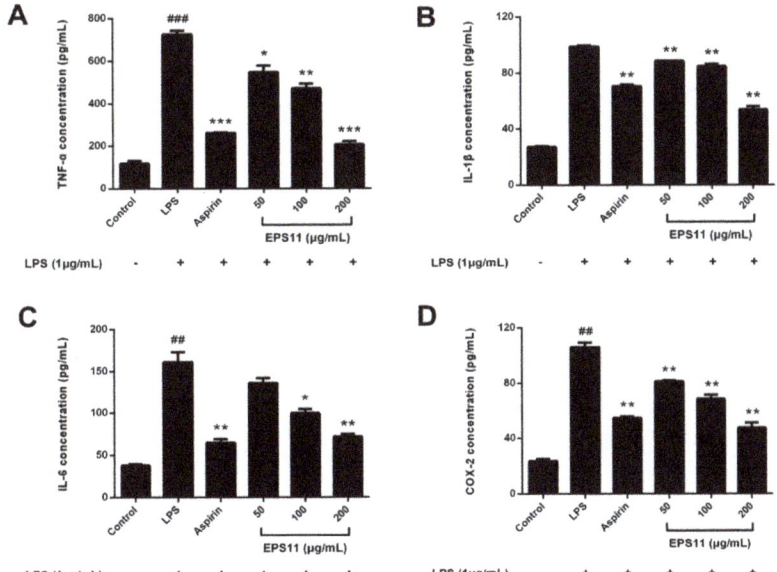

Figure 6. Effects of EPS11 on COX-2, TNF-α, IL-1β, and IL-6 protein expressions in LPS-stimulated RAW 264.7 macrophages. Macrophages cotreated with EPS11 (50, 100, and 200 µg/mL) and LPS (1.0 µg/mL) for 24 h. (**A**) TNF-α, (**B**) IL-1β, (**C**) IL-6, and (**D**) COX-2 determined using ELISA kits. Data presented as mean ± SE (n = 3) from independent experiments. Significance: ## $p < 0.01$, ### $p < 0.001$ vs. control; * $p < 0.05$, ** $p < 0.01$, *** $p < 0.001$ vs. LPS-treated.

2.8. Effects of EPS11 on MAPK Pathways

To explain the mechanism of the anti-inflammatory effects of EPS11 on macrophages, Western blot analysis was applied to assess the effects of EPS11 on MAPK signaling pathways. According to the immunoblots in Figure 7A, phosphorylated P38, JNK, and ERK1/2 were significantly increased in the LPS group. In the test concentrations, EPS11 dramatically depressed the phosphorylated P38, JNK, and ERK1/2, and nonphosphorylated ERK1/2 in a concentration-dependent manner (Figure 7B–D). However, nonphosphorylated P38 and JNK were unchanged in all groups. This indicated that EPS11 may act by inhibiting the phosphorylation of P38, ERK1/2, and JNK, and the expression of ERK1/2 in MAPK pathways.

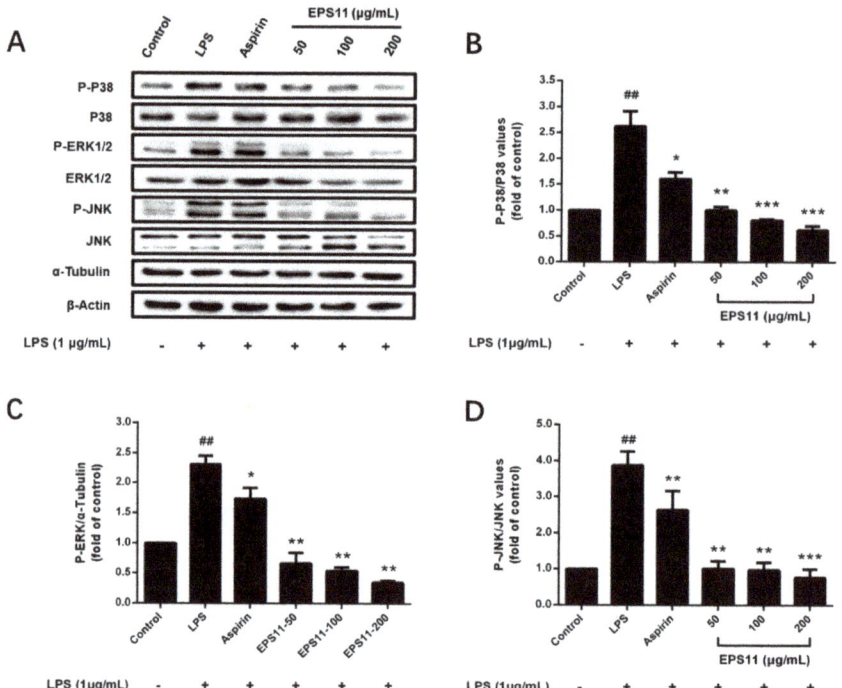

Figure 7. Inhibitory effects of EPS11 on mitogen-activated protein kinase (MAPK) pathway in LPS-stimulated RAW264.7 macrophages. (**A**) Protein-expression levels of P-P38, P38, P-ERK1/2, ERK1/2, P-JNK, and JNK measured by Western blot analysis. Gray value ratios of (**B**) P-P38 to P38, (**C**) P-ERK1/2 to α-tubulin, and (**D**) P-JNK to JNK. Ratio for the control was assigned a value of 1.0. Data presented as mean ± SD ($n = 3$) from independent experiments. Significance: ## $p < 0.01$ vs. control; * $p < 0.05$, ** $p < 0.01$, *** $p < 0.001$ vs. LPS-treated.

2.9. Effects of EPS11 on NF-κB Pathway

IκB and P65 protein levels were determined to unravel the anti-inflammatory mechanism of EPS11 on the NF-κB pathway in RAW264.7 macrophages. As shown in Figure 8A, EPS11 (200 μg/mL) could significantly suppress phosphorylated IκB in LPS-stimulated macrophages, while other concentrations (50 and 100 μg/mL) of EPS11 had no remarkable effect (Figure 8B). Various concentrations of EPS11 (50, 100, and 200 μg/mL) significantly decreased phosphorylated P65 in a concentration-dependent manner, and 200 μg/mL EPS11 completely restrained the phosphorylation of P65 (Figure 8C). The nonphosphorylation of P65 was also almost fully inhibited with EPS11 in the range of 50-100 μg/mL (Figure 8D). This indicated that EPS11 may inhibit the expression or enhance the degradation of NF-κB

P65. Therefore, results revealed that EPS11 suppressed LPS-stimulated NF-κB activation by mainly preventing the phosphorylation or expression of P65.

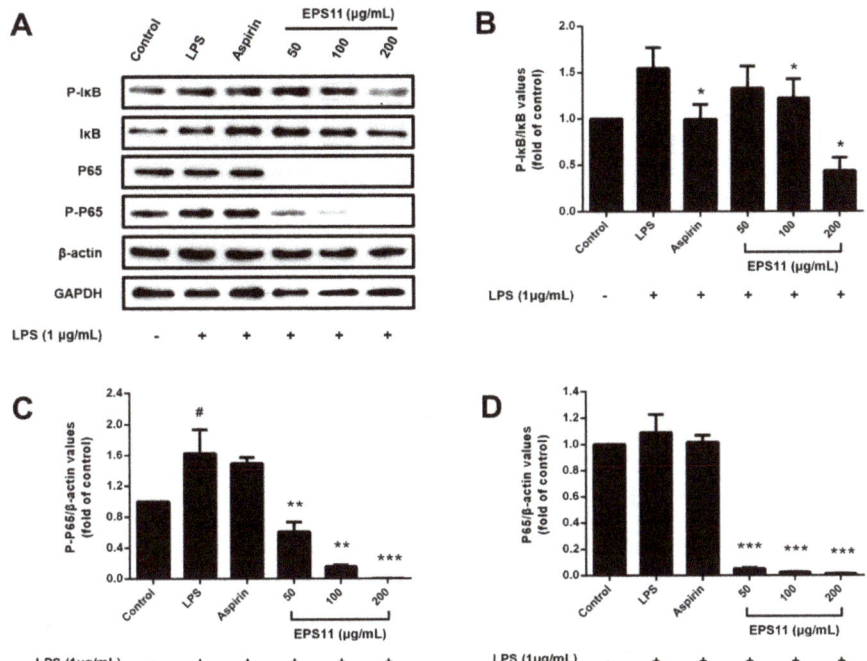

Figure 8. Inhibitory effect of EPS11 on NF-κB pathway in LPS-stimulated RAW264.7 macrophages. (**A**) Protein-expression levels of P-IκB, IκB, P65, and P-P65 measured by Western blot analysis. Gray value ratios of (**B**) p- IκB to IκB, (**C**) P-P65 to β-actin, and (**D**) P65 to β-actin. Ratio for control assigned a value of 1.0. Data presented as mean ± SD (n = 3) from independent experiments. Significance: $^\#$ $p < 0.05$ vs. control; * $p < 0.05$, ** $p < 0.01$, *** $p < 0.001$ vs. LPS-treated.

3. Discussion

In the current study, the inhibitory effects and mechanism of EPS11 against LPS-stimulated inflammatory response were investigated. The results revealed that EPS11 isolated from *Bacillus* sp. BS11 exhibits anti-inflammatory properties, which appeared to be attributable to the inhibition of the activation on MAPK and NF-κB signal pathways in LPS-induced RAW 264.7 macrophages.

It is well known that inhibiting the production of inflammatory cytokines or regulating the balance of key proteins is a possible strategy for treating inflammation [24,25]. Therefore, the generation of NO, IL-1β, IL-6, TNF-α, and COX-2 was determined in LPS-stimulated RAW264.7 macrophages treated with EPS11 (Figures 5 and 6). Data showed that EPS11 can effectively downregulate those inflammatory mediators. The results were consistent with those in a report by Kumar et al., who found that an exopolysaccharide isolated from *Kocuria rosea* strain BS-1 suppressed the release of reactive oxygen species (ROS), NO, TNF-α, and IL-6 from LPS-induced RAW 264.7 macrophages [26]. NO is produced and regulated by Inducible Nitric Oxide Synthase (iNOS), which is activated by immunostimulatory cytokines (such as IL-1β, IL-6, and TNF-α) through the activation of inducible nuclear factors, including NF-κB [23]. The decrease in inflammatory mediators indicated that the activity of inflammation-related signaling pathways was inhibited.

To explore the mechanism of anti-inflammation by EPS11, MAPK signaling pathways were first investigated. MAPK pathways, which mainly included the pathways of P38, ERK1/2, and JNK, could be stimulated by stimuli such as LPS, IL-6, and TNF-α to trigger the inflammation responses. These stimuli could activate ERK, JNK, and P38, and then act on their respective substrates to affect the activity of a variety of transcription factors, thereby regulating the gene expression of various cytokines such as TNF, IL-1, IL-6, and IL-8. In turn, TNF-α, IL-1, and other inflammatory mediators could activate different MAPKs and regulate the production of other inflammatory mediators by promoting or inhibiting the transcription of genes [27,28]. Some natural polysaccharides were reported to inhibit the activation of MAPKs. Wu et al. reported that a sulfated polysaccharide extracted from *Sargassum cristaefolium* could effectively reduce the phosphorylation of P38, ERK, and JNK in LPS-stimulated RAW264.7 macrophages, so as to suppress the expression of iNOS [29]. In this study, EPS11 was found to decrease the phosphorylation of P38, ERK1/2, and JNK in a similar way (Figure 7). This indicated that EPS11 could suppress the activation of MAPK pathways and reduce the intracellular transduction of inflammatory signals, which could downregulate the production of inflammatory mediators by inhibiting the transcription of genes. This might represent a possible mechanism underlying the anti-inflammatory activity of EPS11.

As the downstream-signaling molecules of MAPKs, NF-κB plays a vital role in the progression of inflammation [30]. NF-κB is a dimer protein containing two subunits (P65 and P50) that are tightly inhibited by forming a stable IκB–NF-κB complex in macrophages [31]. IκBα is degraded by the IκB kinase complex (IKK) when macrophages are stimulated by the upstream signal, which allows for the NF-κB proteasome to activate and rapidly translocate into the nucleus [32,33]. In the nucleus, the two subunits (especially P65) bind to a homologous DNA site to start the transcription of relevant genes, which potentially promotes the occurrence and progression of inflammation [34]. The activation of NF-κB in macrophages can promote the expression of proinflammatory cytokines (such as TNF-α, IL-1, and IL-6) and differentiation into the M1 macrophage phenotype [35]. In the present study, EPS11 could significantly block the LPS-stimulated phosphorylation of IκB and P65 (Figure 8). It was proven that inhibiting the phosphorylation of P65 can selectively suppress the expression of many genes associated with inflammatory factors [36]. This suggested that EPS11 not only inhibits the degradation of IκB from the IκB–NF-κB complex, but also prevents the binding of NF-κB to its DNA binding site. Interestingly, EPS11 also inhibited nonphosphorylated P65 in EPS11-treated macrophages. In addition to phosphorylation, another regulatory mechanism (ubiquitination) is activated when NF-κB transports to nucleus. NF-κB is ubiquitinated by the E3 ubiquitin ligase complex and ultimately leads to the degradation of the NF-κB heterodimer protein [37,38]. Ubiquitination is regulated by deubiquitinase ubiquitin specific protease-7 (USP7), which specifically requires P65 as the substrate. The inactivation of USP7 activity results in the reduced expression of target genes and P65 degradation [39]. This implied that EPS11 may suppress the expression of P65 by enhancing its ubiquitination and degradation. Therefore, it is possible that EPS11 inhibited the phosphorylation and promoted the ubiquitination of NF-κB P65 to decrease the transcription and expression of inflammatory mediators and prevent macrophages from differentiating into the M1 phenotype.

4. Experiments and Methods

4.1. Materials and Reagents

Bacillus sp. BS11 was isolated from marine mud samples collected near the Yap Trench (1143 m deep) in the tropical Western Pacific (139°3802′ E, 11°44162′ N); the RAW 264.7 macrophage line was purchased from Macrophage Resource Center, Shanghai Institute of Life Sciences, Chinese Academy of Sciences (Shanghai, China); 1-phenyl-3-methyl-5-pyrazolone (PMP) was purchased from Sigma-Aldrich (St. Louis, MO, USA); Dulbecco's Modified Eagle's Medium (DMEM)/high-glucose medium was purchased from HyClone (Logan, UT, USA); lipopolysaccharides (LPS) and aspirin were purchased from Yuanye (Shanghai, China); 3-(4, 5-dimethylthiazol-2-yl)-2, 5-diphenyltetrazolium bromide (MTT) reagent and dimethyl sulfoxide (DMSO) were purchased from Sigma-Aldrich (St. Louis, MO, USA); fetal bovine serum (FBS) was purchased from Gibco Life Technologies (Grand Island, NY, USA);

ELISA kit for the analysis of cyclooxygenase (COX-2), TNF-α, IL-1β, and IL-6 production was obtained from AndHider (Qingdao, Shandong, China); Griess reagent, NG-monomethyl-L-arginine, monoacetate salt (L-NMMA), and horseradish peroxidase (HRP)-conjugated goat antimouse IgG secondary antibodies were purchased from Beyotime (Nantong, Jiangsu, China); antibodies to ERK, phosphorylated ERK (P-ERK), JNK, phosphorylated JNK (p-JNK), P38, phosphorylated P38 (P-P38), IκBα, phosphorylated IκBα (p-IκBα), P65, phosphorylated P65 (P-P65), and β-actin were purchased from Santa Cruz (Dallas, TX, USA); antibodies to GADPH and α-tubulin were purchased from Abcam (Cambridge, MA, USA); HRP-conjugated goat antirabbit IgG secondary antibodies were purchased from Affinity (Chicago, IL, USA).

4.2. Extraction and Purification of EPS11 from Bacillus sp.BS11

The pure culture of marine *Bacillus* sp.BS11 was inoculated to a 2216E medium (0.5% tryptone, 0.1% yeast extract powder, and 1% sucrose; pH = 7.5) in a proportion of 0.1% (v/v) and cultured at 28 °C and 140 RPM for 24 h. To obtain the precipitation of the crude polysaccharide, the supernatant, which was obtained by centrifugation (8000 RPM, 20 min) of the fermentation liquid, was precipitated with triple alcohol by volume. Precipitation was again dispersed in pure water, and mixed with Sevag's reagent (chloroform:N-butyl alcohol = 5:1, v/v) in a ratio of 4:1 to remove the proteins [40]. The crude polysaccharide was obtained with the dialysis (MWCO: 8.0 kD), concentration, and lyophilization of the supernatant.

To obtain a homogeneous polysaccharide, diethylaminoethyl cellulose (DEAE) Fast Flow anion-exchange column was devoted to purifying the crude polysaccharide using 50 mmol/L NaCl with 20 mmol/L Tris-HCl buffer (pH = 9.0) and a linear gradient eluent (from 50 to 500 mmol/L NaCl solution with 20 mmol/L Tris-HCl buffer). The fractions were recorded and collected by AKTA Purifier (GE Healthcare, USA). The collected polysaccharide fractions continued to be purified with a HiLoad™ 16/600 Superdex™ 200 gel chromatographic column (GE Healthcare, USA), which used 150 mmol/L NaCl and 20 mmol/L Tris-HCl buffer (pH = 9.0) as the mobile phase. The final polysaccharide fraction (EPS11) was collected, dialyzed, and lyophilized.

4.3. Determination of Physical and Chemical Properties

Total EPS11 content was determined by the sulfuric acid-phenol method, which uses Man as standard to draw the standard curve. The protein content was determined using a bicinchoninic acid (BCA) kit (Solarbio, Beijing, China). Moisture content was measured by the ambient-pressure-drying method, which needs the sample to be dried to a constant weight. The amino acid composition of EPS11 was determined using an automatic amino acid analyzer (L-8500A, Hitachi, Japan).

The monosaccharide composition of EPS11 was measured by the method of precolumn derivation RP-HPLC [41,42]. EPS11 (5.0 mg/mL) was hydrolyzed in a sealed tube with conditions of 2.0 mol/L trifluoroacetic acid (TFA), 105 °C, and 4 h. The TFA was neutralized by NaOH solution. Then, the hydrolysate or monosaccharide standard was derivatized with 0.5 mol/L PMP-methanol (120 µL) and 0.3 mol/L NaOH (100 µL) for 1 h at 70 °C. The reaction liquid was extracted by chloroform three times after it was neutralized with HCl. The derivatives were filtered with a micron membrane filter (0.22 µm) to perform HPLC analysis under the given chromatographic conditions (Table 4). The molar ratio of the monosaccharides was calculated on the basis of the peak area and relative molecular mass of each monosaccharide.

Table 4. Chromatographic conditions of monosaccharide composition.

	Parameters
Mobile phase	0.1 mol/L phosphate-buffered saline (PBS; pH 6.8): acetonitrile = 83:17 (v/v, %)
Chromatographic column	ZORBAX SB-AQ C18 column (4.6 × 250 mm, 5 µm)
Temperature	30 °C
Flow rate	0.8 mL/min
Detector	Variable-wavelength detector (VWD; 245 nm)

High-performance gel-permeation chromatography (HPGPC) was carried out to determine the molecular weight of EPS11 with a refractive-index detector. EPS11 solution (5 mg/mL) was eluted by 0.1 mol/L Na_2SO_4 through a SHODEX SUGAR KS-804 (7.8 × 300 nm) column (SHODEX, Tokyo, Japan). Column temperature and flow rate were set as 35 °C and 0.5 mL/min, respectively. The calculation of the molecular weight was according to the standard curve that was plotted with the retention time and the molecular weight of dextran (5250, 9750, 13,150, 36,800, 64,650, 135,350, and 300,600 Da).

4.4. Infrared Spectrum

The FT–IR spectrum was recorded on a Nicolet iS 10 FT–IR spectrometer (Thermo Fisher, Waltham, MA, USA) in the range of 400–4000 cm^{-1}.

4.5. Protein Identification by LC-MS/MS

EPS11 solid was added to a trypsin buffer (6μg Trypsin in 40μL NH_4HCO_3 buffer), and the mixtures were incubated at 37 °C for18 h. The peptides were desalted using C18 StageTip (Thermo Scientific) and separated using an EASY-nLC 1200 Nano UHPLC system (Thermo Fisher, Waltham, MA, USA) equipped with a Trap Column (100 μm 20 mm, 5 μm, C18, Dr. Maisch GmbH, Ammerbuch-Entringen, Germany). The sample was injected and separated by a chromatographic column (75 μm 150 mm, 3 μm, C18, Dr. Maisch GmbH) at a flow rate of 300 nl/min. The liquid phase separation gradient is as follows: Buffer solution A is 0.1% formic acid aqueous solution, B is 0.1% formic acid, acetonitrile and water mixture solution (acetonitrile: 95%). 0–3 min, 2–7% B; 3–48 min, 7–35% B; 48–53 min, 35–90% B; 53–60 min, 90% B. Data-dependent acquisition (DDA) mass spectrometry was performed with a Q-Exactive HFX mass spectrometer (Thermo Scientific) after peptide separation. The analysis time was 60 min, detection mode: positive ion, parent ion scanning range: 300–1800 m/z, primary mass spectrometric resolution: 70,000 m/z 200. Secondary mass spectrogram of 20 parent ions with the highest intensity was acquired after each full scan. The software MaxQuant1.6.1.0 and Uniprot Protein Database were used to analyze the mass spectrometry database.

4.6. Macrophage Culture and Treatment

RAW 264.7 macrophages were incubated in a DMEM/high-glucose culture medium that was mixed with 10% FBS and 1% antibiotics (100 U/mL penicillin and 100 U/mL streptomycin) and placed in a CO_2 incubator (5% CO_2, 37 °C). When they had grown to 80% of the area of the culture flask, the macrophages were washed down and planted in 96- or 6-well plates with cell density of 5×10^3 cells/well, and incubated for 24 h. Then, different concentrations of EPS11 (0–200 μg/mL) or mixed with LPS (1.0 μg/mL) were added to the corresponding wells for 24 h. L-NMMA (50 μmol/L) or aspirin (200 μg/mL) was used as the positive drug, and untreated macrophages were used as the control group.

4.7. Assessment of Cell Viability

The effect of EPS11 on the viability of RAW 264.7 macrophages was evaluated by MTT assay [43]. To rule out the potential influences of drugs on cell viability, the macrophages were treated by different concentrations of EPS11 (6.25, 12.5, 25, 50, 80, 100, and 200 μg/mL) or with LPS (1.0 μg/mL) in 96-well plates for 24 h. FBS-free medium (100 μL) and 5.0 mg/mL MTT stock solution (10 μL) were immediately added to each well and incubated for 4 h to form the formazan. Then, the supernatants were carefully discarded, and DMSO (50 μL) was added to entirely dissolve the formazan. The absorbance was measured at 570 nm. Cell viability is presented in the form of percentage contrasted with the control group.

4.8. Active Fraction Appraisal

As EPS11 is a proteoglycan, it is not known which part performs the anti-inflammatory activity. To identify the active fraction, EPS11 (200 µg/mL) was treated with proteinase K (50 µg/mL) and NaIO4 (15 mmol/L), respectively. Then, the LPS-induced RAW264.7 macrophages were incubated with EPS11 that was treated in two different ways. The levels of NO production were detected to evaluate anti-inflammatory activity of each fraction.

4.9. Determination of NO Production

NO concentration in the supernatant was measured using the Griess reagent [44]. RAW264.7 macrophages were treated by different concentrations of EPS11 (6.25, 12.5, 25, 50, 100, and 200 µg/mL) or with LPS (1.0 µg/mL) in 96-well plates for 24 h. Cell-culture supernatants (50 µL) were sucked out into a new plate, and Griess reagents I (50 µL) and II (50 µL) were added in each well. The NO concentration was calculated according to the standard curve, which was measured at 540 nm.

4.10. COX-2 and Cytokine Assays

RAW264.7 macrophages were cotreated by various concentrations of EPS11 (50, 100, and 200 µg/mL) and LPS (1.0 µg/mL) in 6-well plates for 24 h. The cell-culture supernatants in each well were collected and centrifuged to measure the levels of COX-2 and inflammatory cytokines (TNF-α, IL-1β, and IL-6) using commercial ELISA kits according to operating instructions.

4.11. Western Blot Analysis

RAW 264.7 macrophages were cotreated by EPS11 (50, 100, and 200 µg/mL) and LPS (1.0 µg/mL) in 6-well plates for 24 h. Then, the total proteins of the macrophages were extracted by 100 µL RIPA lysis buffer (G-CLONE, Beijing, China). The protein content of every group was determined by BCA protein assay kit (Solarbio, Beijing, China). The total proteins were corrected to equivalents and denatured with loading buffer. The target proteins were separated by SDS-polyacrylamide gel electrophoresis (SDS-PAGE) and transferred to a nitrocellulose-filter (NC) membrane. Then, the membrane was sealed with 5% skim milk, hybridized with primary antibodies, and incubated with a secondary antibody in sequence. Enhanced chemiluminescence (Vazyme, Nanjing, China) was applied to detect protein blots using a ChemiDoc MP system (Bio-Rad Laboratories, Hercules, CA, USA). The relative grayscale of the protein band was calculated by using Image J v.1.52a (National Institutes of Health, Bethesda, MD, USA).

4.12. Statistical Analysis

The statistical analysis was performed using Prism 6 (version 6.01, GraphPad Software, San Diego, CA, USA). All data are presented as the average value ± SD from at least three independent experiments. The significance was analyzed between the two groups using an unpaired t-test. A p value < 0.05 was considered to be the level of statistical significance (* $p < 0.05$, ** $p < 0.01$, *** $p < 0.001$).

5. Conclusions

The current study suggested that marine bacterial proteoglycan (EPS11) exhibited strong anti-inflammatory activity. This could significantly decrease the generation of NO, COX-2, TNF-α, IL-1β, and IL-6 through suppressing the phosphorylation of P38, ERK1/2, and JNK in MAPK pathways, and the expression of NF-κB P65 in LPS-stimulated RAW 264.7 macrophages. Moreover, EPS11 may mainly inhibit the NF-κB pathway to execute this anti-inflammatory effect. Future studies are expected to confirm the anti-inflammatory effect in inflammatory animal models, and ultimately demonstrate the potential application of EPS11 in the treatment of inflammatory diseases.

Author Contributions: Q.W., C.S., and Q.Z. brought up the assumption and designed the experiments. Q.W. carried out most of the experiments. W.L. separated and purified the EPS11. Y.Y. helped to perform the study of anti-inflammatory activity in vitro. Q.W., Y.Y. and C.S. analyzed the data. Q.W. and Q.Z. prepared the figures and wrote the paper. All authors have read and agreed to the published version of the manuscript.

Funding: This research was funded by the China Ocean Mineral Resources R&D Association, grant number DY135-B2-14.

Conflicts of Interest: The authors declare no conflict of interest.

References

1. Naik, S.R.; Wala, S.M. Inflammation, Allergy and Asthma, Complex Immune Origin Diseases: Mechanisms and Therapeutic Agents. *Recent Pat. Inflamm. Allergy Drug Discov.* **2013**, *7*, 62–95. [CrossRef]
2. Dickens, A.M.; Tovar-Y-Romo, L.B.; Yoo, S.W.; Trout, A.L.; Bae, M.; Kanmogne, M.; Megra, B.; Williams, D.W.; Witwer, K.W.; Gacias, M. Astrocyte-shed extracellular vesicles regulate the peripheral leukocyte response to inflammatory brain lesions. *Sci. Signal.* **2017**, *10*, eaai7696. [CrossRef] [PubMed]
3. Simmonds, R.E.; Foxwell, B.M. Signalling, inflammation and arthritis: NF-kappaB and its relevance to arthritis and inflammation. *Rheumatology* **2008**, *47*, 584–590. [CrossRef] [PubMed]
4. Mantovani, A.; Allavena, P.; Sica, A.; Balkwill, F. Cancer-related inflammation. *Nature* **2008**, *454*, 436–444. [CrossRef] [PubMed]
5. Willerson, J.T.; Ridker, P.M. Inflammation as a cardiovascular risk factor. *Circulation* **2004**, *109* (Suppl. 1), II2–II10. [CrossRef] [PubMed]
6. Weiner, H.L. Multiple Sclerosis Is an Inflammatory T-Cell–Mediated Autoimmune Disease. *Arch. Neurol.* **2004**, *61*, 1613–1615. [CrossRef] [PubMed]
7. de Araujo Boleti, A.P.; de Oliveira Flores, T.M.; Moreno, S.E.; Anjos, L.D.; Mortari, M.R.; Migliolo, L. Neuroinflammation: An overview of neurodegenerative and metabolic diseases and of biotechnological studies. *Neurochem. Int.* **2020**, *136*, 104714. [CrossRef]
8. Kwak, B.; Mulhaupt, F.; Myit, S.; Mach, F. Statins as a newly recognized type of immunomodulator. *Nat. Med.* **2000**, *6*, 1399–1402. [CrossRef]
9. Kim, H.; Lee, T.H.; Hwang, Y.S.; Bang, M.A.; Shong, M. Methimazole As an Antioxidant and Immunomodulator in Thyroid Cells: Mechanisms Involving Interferon-γ Signaling and H_2O_2 Scavenging. *Mol. Pharmacol.* **2001**, *60*, 972–980. [CrossRef]
10. Fay, A.P.; Moreira, R.B.; Nunes Filho, P.R.S.; Albuquerque, C.; Barrios, C.H. The management of immune-related adverse events associated with immune checkpoint blockade. *Expert Rev. Qual. Life Cancer Care* **2016**, *1*, 89–97. [CrossRef]
11. Geng, L.H.; Hu, W.C.; Liu, Y.J.; Wang, J.; Zhang, Q.B. A heteropolysaccharide from Saccharina japonica with immunomodulatory effect on RAW 264.7 cells. *Carbohydr. Polym.* **2018**, *201*, 557–565. [CrossRef] [PubMed]
12. Fang, Q.; Wang, J.F.; Zha, X.Q.; Cui, S.H.; Cao, L.; Luo, J.P. Immunomodulatory activity on macrophage of a purified polysaccharide extracted from Laminaria japonica. *Carbohydr. Polym.* **2015**, *134*, 66–73. [CrossRef] [PubMed]
13. Nie, C.Z.P.; Zhu, P.L.; Ma, S.P.; Wang, M.C.; Hu, Y.D. Purification, characterization and immunomodulatory activity of polysaccharides from stem lettuce. *Carbohydr. Polym.* **2018**, *188*, 236–242. [CrossRef] [PubMed]
14. Beutler, B. Innate immunity: An overview. *Mol. Immunol.* **2004**, *40*, 845–859. [CrossRef]
15. Palsson-McDermott, E.M.; O'Neill, L.A. Signal transduction by the lipopolysaccharide receptor, Toll-like receptor-4. *Immunology* **2004**, *113*, 153–162. [CrossRef]
16. Lee, J.S.; Kwon, D.S.; Lee, K.R.; Park, J.M.; Ha, S.J.; Hong, E.K. Mechanism of macrophage activation induced by polysaccharide from Cordyceps militaris culture broth. *Carbohydr. Polym.* **2015**, *120*, 29–37. [CrossRef]
17. Hunter, M.; Wang, Y.; Eubank, T.; Baran, C.; Nana-Sinkam, P.; Marsh, C. Survival of monocytes and macrophages and their role in health and disease. *Front. Biosci. J. Virtual Libr.* **2009**, *14*, 4079. [CrossRef]
18. Mandal, P.; Pratt, B.T.; Barnes, M.; McMullen, M.R.; Nagy, L.E. Molecular mechanism for adiponectin-dependent M2 macrophage polarization: Link between the metabolic and innate immune activity of full-length adiponectin. *J. Biol. Chem.* **2011**, *286*, 13460–13469. [CrossRef]
19. Yoo, M.S.; Shin, J.S.; Choi, H.E.; Cho, Y.W.; Bang, M.H.; Baek, N.I.; Lee, K.T. Fucosterol isolated from Undaria pinnatifida inhibits lipopolysaccharide-induced production of nitric oxide and pro-inflammatory cytokines via the inactivation of nuclear factor-kappaB and p38 mitogen-activated protein kinase in RAW264.7 macrophages. *Food Chem.* **2012**, *135*, 967–975. [CrossRef]

20. Van den Bossche, J.; O'Neill, L.A.; Menon, D. Macrophage Immunometabolism: Where Are We (Going)? *Trends Immunol.* **2017**, *38*, 395–406. [CrossRef]
21. Cao, R.B.; Jin, W.H.; Shan, Y.Q.; Wang, J.; Liu, G.; Kuang, S.; Sun, C.M. Marine Bacterial Polysaccharide EPS11 Inhibits Cancer Cell Growth via Blocking Cell Adhesion and Stimulating Anoikis. *Mar. Drugs* **2018**, *16*, 85. [CrossRef] [PubMed]
22. Wang, J.; Liu, G.; Ma, W.P.; Lu, Z.X.; Sun, C.M. Marine Bacterial Polysaccharide EPS11 Inhibits Cancer Cell Growth and Metastasis via Blocking Cell Adhesion and Attenuating Filiform Structure Formation. *Mar. Drugs* **2019**, *17*, 50. [CrossRef] [PubMed]
23. Aktan, F. iNOS-mediated nitric oxide production and its regulation. *Life Sci.* **2004**, *75*, 639–653. [CrossRef] [PubMed]
24. Du, B.; Lin, C.Y.; Bian, Z.X.; Xu, B.J. An insight into anti-inflammatory effects of fungal beta-glucans. *Trends Food Sci. Technol.* **2015**, *41*, 49–59. [CrossRef]
25. Zhu, F.M.; Du, B.; Xu, B.J. Anti-inflammatory effects of phytochemicals from fruits, vegetables, and food legumes: A review. *Crit. Rev. Food Sci. Nutr.* **2018**, *58*, 1260–1270. [CrossRef]
26. Kumar, C.G.; Sujitha, P. Kocuran, an exopolysaccharide isolated from Kocuria rosea strain BS-1 and evaluation of its in vitro immunosuppression activities. *Enzyme Microb. Technol.* **2014**, *55*, 113–120. [CrossRef]
27. Branger, J.; van den Blink, B.; Weijer, S.; Madwed, J.; Bos, C.L.; Gupta, A.; Yong, C.L.; Polmar, S.H.; Olszyna, D.P.; Hack, C.E. Anti-inflammatory effects of a p38 mitogen-activated protein kinase inhibitor during human endotoxemia. *J. Immunol.* **2002**, *168*, 4070. [CrossRef]
28. Uto, T.; Fujii, M.; Hou, D.X. 6-(Methylsulfinyl)hexyl isothiocyanate suppresses inducible nitric oxide synthase expression through the inhibition of Janus kinase 2-mediated JNK pathway in lipopolysaccharide-activated murine macrophages. *Biochem. Pharmacol.* **2005**, *70*, 1211–1221. [CrossRef]
29. Wu, G.J.; Shiu, S.M.; Hsieh, M.C.; Tsai, G.J. Anti-inflammatory activity of a sulfated polysaccharide from the brown alga Sargassum cristaefolium. *Food Hydrocoll.* **2016**, *53*, 16–23. [CrossRef]
30. Paunovic, V.; Harnett, M.M. Mitogen-activated protein kinases as therapeutic targets for rheumatoid arthritis. *Drugs* **2013**, *73*, 101–115. [CrossRef]
31. Wong, D.; Teixeira, A.; Oikonomopoulos, S.; Humburg, P.; Lone, I.N.; Saliba, D.; Siggers, T.; Bulyk, M.; Angelov, D.; Dimitrov, S.; et al. Extensive characterization of NF-kappaB binding uncovers non-canonical motifs and advances the interpretation of genetic functional traits. *Genome Biol.* **2011**, *12*, R70. [CrossRef] [PubMed]
32. Pan, M.H.; Lin-Shiau, S.Y.; Lin, J.K. Comparative studies on the suppression of nitric oxide synthase by curcumin and its hydrogenated metabolites through down-regulation of IκB kinase and NFκB activation in macrophages. *Biochem. Pharmacol.* **2000**, *60*, 1665–1676. [CrossRef]
33. Thompson, J.E.; Phillips, R.J.; Erdjument-Bromage, H.; Tempst, P.; Ghosh, S. IκB-β regulates the persistent response in a biphasic activation of NF-κB. *Cell* **1995**, *80*, 573–582. [CrossRef]
34. Sen, R. Inducibility of kappa immunoglobulin enhancer-binding protein Nf-kappa B by a posttranslational mechanism. *Cell* **1986**, *47*, 921–928. [CrossRef]
35. Liu, T.; Zhang, L.; Joo, D.; Sun, S.C. NF-κB signaling in inflammation. *Signal Transduct. Target. Ther.* **2017**, *2*, 17023. [CrossRef]
36. Nowak, D.E.; Tian, B.; Jamaluddin, M.; Boldogh, I.; Vergara, L.A.; Choudhary, S.; Brasier, A.R. RelA Ser276 phosphorylation is required for activation of a subset of NF-kappaB-dependent genes by recruiting cyclin-dependent kinase 9/cyclin T1 complexes. *Mol. Cell. Biol.* **2008**, *28*, 3623–3638. [CrossRef]
37. Mao, X.; Gluck, N.; Li, D.; Maine, G.N.; Li, H.; Zaidi, I.W.; Repaka, A.; Mayo, M.W.; Burstein, E. GCN5 is a required cofactor for a ubiquitin ligase that targets NF-kappaB/RelA. *Genes Dev.* **2009**, *23*, 849–861. [CrossRef]
38. Saccani, S.; Marazzi, I.; Beg, A.A.; Natoli, G. Degradation of promoter-bound p65/RelA is essential for the prompt termination of the nuclear factor kappaB response. *J. Exp. Med.* **2004**, *200*, 107–113. [CrossRef]
39. Colleran, A.; Collins, P.E.; O'Carroll, C.; Ahmed, A.; Mao, X.; Mcmanus, B.; Kiely, P.A.; Burstein, E.; Carmody, R.J. Deubiquitination of NF-κB by Ubiquitin-Specific Protease-7 promotes transcription. *Proc. Natl. Acad. Sci. USA* **2013**, *110*, 618–623. [CrossRef]
40. Sun, S.; Li, K.J.; Xiao, L.; Lei, Z.F.; Zhang, Z.Y. Characterization of polysaccharide from Helicteres angustifolia L. and its immunomodulatory activities on macrophages RAW264.7. *Biomed. Pharmacother.* **2019**, *109*, 262–270. [CrossRef]

41. Dai, J.; Wu, Y.; Chen, S.W.; Zhu, S.; Yin, H.P.; Wang, M.; Tang, J. Sugar compositional determination of polysaccharides from Dunaliella salina by modified RP-HPLC method of precolumn derivatization with 1-phenyl-3-methyl-5-pyrazolone. *Carbohydr. Polym.* **2010**, *82*, 629–635. [CrossRef]
42. Wu, J.D.; Zhao, X.; Ren, L.; Xue, Y.T.; Li, C.X.; Yu, G.L.; Guan, H.S. Determination of M/G ratio of propylene glycol alginate sodium sulfate by HPLC with pre-column derivatization. *Carbohydr. Polym.* **2014**, *104*, 23–28. [CrossRef] [PubMed]
43. Tahmourespour, A.; Ahmadi, A.; Fesharaki, M. The anti-tumor activity of exopolysaccharides from Pseudomonas strains against HT-29 colorectal cancer cell line. *Int. J. Biol. Macromol.* **2020**, *149*, 1072–1076. [CrossRef] [PubMed]
44. Zhao, X.T.; Hou, P.L.; Xin, H.J.; Zhang, Y.Q.; Zhou, A.M.; Lai, C.J.S.; Xie, J.B. A glucogalactomanan polysaccharide isolated from Agaricus bisporus causes an inflammatory response via the ERK/MAPK and IkappaB/NFkappaB pathways in macrophages. *Int. J. Biol. Macromol.* **2020**, *151*, 1067–1073. [CrossRef] [PubMed]

Publisher's Note: MDPI stays neutral with regard to jurisdictional claims in published maps and institutional affiliations.

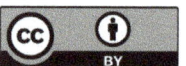

© 2020 by the authors. Licensee MDPI, Basel, Switzerland. This article is an open access article distributed under the terms and conditions of the Creative Commons Attribution (CC BY) license (http://creativecommons.org/licenses/by/4.0/).

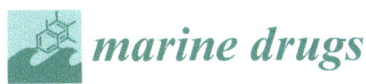

Article

Particulate Matter-Induced Inflammation/Oxidative Stress in Macrophages: Fucosterol from *Padina boryana* as a Potent Protector, Activated via NF-κB/MAPK Pathways and Nrf2/HO-1 Involvement

Thilina U. Jayawardena [1], K. K. Asanka Sanjeewa [1], Hyo-Geun Lee [1], D. P. Nagahawatta [1], Hye-Won Yang [1], Min-Cheol Kang [2,*] and You-Jin Jeon [1,3,*]

1. Department of Marine Life Sciences, Jeju National University, Jeju 690-756, Korea; tujayawardena@jejunu.ac.kr (T.U.J.); asanka@jejunu.ac.kr (K.K.A.S.); hyogeunlee92@jejunu.ac.kr (H.-G.L.); pramuditha1992@jejunu.ac.kr (D.P.N.); koty221@naver.com (H.-W.Y.)
2. Research Group of Process Engineering, Korea Food Research Institute, Jeollabuk-do 55365, Korea
3. Marine Science Institute, Jeju National University, Jeju 63333, Korea
* Correspondence: mckang@kfri.re.kr (M.-C.K.); youjinj@jejunu.ac.kr (Y.-J.J.); Tel.: +82-064-754-3475 (Y.-J.J.)

Received: 3 November 2020; Accepted: 8 December 2020; Published: 9 December 2020

Abstract: Fucosterol is a phytosterol that is abundant in marine brown algae and is a renowned secondary metabolite. However, its ability to protect macrophages against particulate matter (PM) has not been clarified with regard to inflammation; thus, this study aimed to illustrate the above. *Padina boryana*, a brown algae that is widespread in Indo–Pacific waters, was applied in the isolation of fucosterol. Isolation was conducted using silica open columns, while identification was assisted with gas chromatography-mass spectroscopy (GC-MS) and NMR. Elevated levels of PM led the research objectives toward the implementation of it as a stimulant. Both inflammation and oxidative stress were caused due the fact of its effect. RAW 264.7 macrophages were used as a model system to evaluate the process. It was apparent that the increased NO production levels, due to the PM, were mediated through the inflammatory mediators, such as inducible nitric oxide synthase (iNOS), cyclooxygenase-2 (COX-2) and pro-inflammatory cytokines (i.e., interleukin-6 (IL-6), interleukin-1 (IL-1β) and tumor necrosis factor-α (TNF-α), including prostaglandin E2 (PGE$_2$)). Further, investigations provided solid evidence regarding the involvement of NF-κB and mitogen-activated protein kinases (MAPKs) in the process. Oxidative stress/inflammation which are inseparable components of the cellular homeostasis were intersected through the Nrf2/HO-1 pathway. Conclusively, fucosterol is a potent protector against PM-induced inflammation in macrophages and hence be utilized as natural product secondary metabolite in a sustainable manner.

Keywords: *Padina boryana*; RAW 264.7 macrophages; Nrf2/HO-1; MAPK; NF-κB

1. Introduction

The destruction of the ecological environment is being contributed to by various factors such as biologically hazardous and chemical waste. Over the past decade, ambient air pollution through vehicle emission dust and industrial emissions has increased. It has been reported that air pollution is the world's single largest environmental health risk [1]. Airborne particulate matter (PM) is associated with various health risks including respiratory disorders, allergic reactions, cardiovascular diseases and dermal diseases. PM has become a major concern globally, in particular in the East Asia region including China, Korea and Japan. Beijing is considered as one of the most heaviest air polluted cities in the world [2]. Though anthropogenic sources are contributing towards this, a major natural contributor is the particulate matter originating during the spring season in the Loess Plateau, the desert regions of

Mongolia and northwest China. Lee et al. (2015) reported that emissions released by China were much smaller compared with non-anthropogenic sources [3].

PM is a complex mixture of biological materials (e.g., pollen, micro-organisms), metallic ions, organic matter and poly-aromatic hydrocarbons. The inorganic composition of fine dust was characterized by Maxwell et al. (2004) using Asian dust, and the main components were reported as water-soluble mineral dust including Mg^{2+} and Ca^{2+}. Further, fine-particle negative ions remained as nitrate (NO_3^-) and sulfate (SO_4^{2-}) associated with ammonium (NH_4^+) or potassium (K^+) [4]. Factors which influence the toxicity of PM were reported by Harrison and Yin (2000) as being bulk chemical composition, trace element content, strong acid content, sulfate content and particle size distribution [5]. Lv et al. (2016) systematically analyzed PM 2.5 Beijing urban fine dust and its sources descriptively with environmental impacts [6]. Particulate matter is generally composed of coarse and fine fractions. The coarse fraction consists mainly of natural sources such as re-suspended dust and biological material (e.g., pollen, bacteria), whereas the fine particles, which are less than 2.5 μm, are dominated by anthropogenic emissions [7].

Earlier reports have indicated that the metal content and its acidity, specifically transition metals, interfere with host defense mechanisms and cause inflammation [8,9]. In vitro PM pollution studies have exhibited cytotoxicity, oxygen radical formation and cytokine release, signifying the effect of particulate pollution in inflammatory disorders [10,11]. Shukla et al. (1999) reported on the effect of fine particulate matter inhalation and nuclear factor kappa-B (NF-κB)-related inflammatory activation in pulmonary epithelial cells [12]. Similarly, Zhao et al. (2016) reported on the effect of fine dust in inflammatory pathway activation through reactive oxygen species (ROS)-dependent mechanisms [13]. ROS plays an important role in the elimination of microbes inside the lungs, though the over production of ROS results in oxidative stress due to the fact that live cells are damaged, leading to internal disorders. Respiratory diseases, excessive inflammation and oxidative stress are reported as the major causes [14,15].

During their lifespan, marine algae are exposed to extreme conditions. They face high oxygen concentrations, intense light, UV radiation and stress. Due to the fact of their rich bioactive components, stressful conditions can be overcome successfully [16]. Earlier studies focused on the different bioactive components from brown algae such as fucoxanthin [16], chromenes [17] and diphlorethohydroxycarmalol [18].

Padina boryana is a brown algae species that is widespread in warm Indo–Pacific waters. This species has been the subject of study on several previous occasions. Fernando et al. (2018) used the carbohydrase assisted extraction for *P. boryana* and evaluated its antioxidant and anti-inflammatory potentials briefly [19]. Fucoidan from this species has been widely studied for its structure and anticancer activity by Usoltseva et al. (2017) [20].

Fucosterol is phytosterol, apparently abundant in brown algae, and was first identified in its pure form by Heilbron et al. (1934) who published an article highlighting its potentials [21]. Its various properties have been reported vividly on different occasions. The antioxidant effects of fucosterol were reported using *Pelvetia siliquosa* [22]. Its anti-inflammatory properties against LPS-stimulated conditions were earlier reported by Jung et al. (2013) using brown algae, *Elsenia bicyclis* [23]. The anti-osteoporotic effect was evaluated using fucosterol derived from *Undaria pinnatifida* [24]. Fernando et al. (2019) studied and reported on the potential of fucosterol to inhibit particulate matter-induced inflammation and oxidative stress in the alveolar cell line A549 [25].

This study aimed to isolate fucosterol from the brown algae *P. boryana* and to evaluate its anti-inflammatory properties on PM-induced RAW 264.7 macrophages. Pure compound fucosterol identification was assisted by nuclear magnetic resonance spectroscopy (NMR) and gas chromatography-mass spectroscopy (GC-MS) data. The preliminary studies revealed its potential to inhibit PM-induced inflammation. Hence, further studies were conducted to confirm its activity using RT-qPCR techniques for gene expression analysis and Western blotting as well as enzyme-linked immunosorbent assay (ELISA) techniques. The activity was anticipated to occur via the mitogen-activated protein kinase (MAPK) and NF-κB pathways. Further, we elevated our studies to the level of oxidative stress-related protein expression analysis. To the best of our knowledge, this is the first report with regard to the assessment of fucosterol on particulate matter-induced inflammation in RAW 264.7 macrophages.

2. Results

2.1. Characterization of Particulate Matter

Certified reference material No. 28; China fine dust particulate matter (PM) was used for the experiments. Mori et al. (2008) reported the detailed procedures for the collection of particulate matter through mechanical vibration and the chemical characterization [26]. Scanning electron microscope imaging was conducted in order to evaluate the particle size and distribution (Figure 1a). It was evident that the majority of particles possessed a diameter less than 5 μm. Furthermore, we referred to the data provided by the National Institute for Environmental Studies (NIES), Ibaraki, Japan, and supply them below in Figure 1b–d for reference.

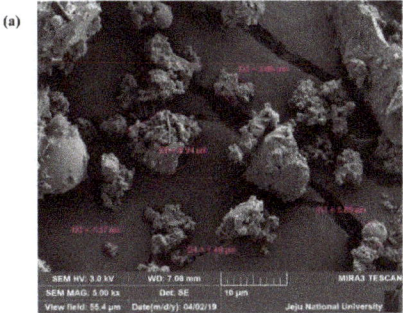
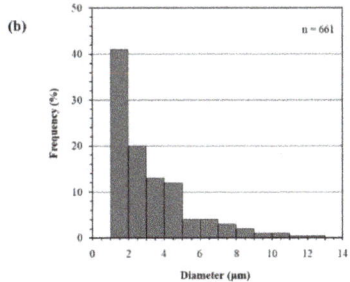

(c)

Element	Mass fraction (ppm)
Na	7960.0 ± 650.0
Mg	14000.0 ± 600.0
Al	50400.0 ± 1000.0
K	13700.0 ± 600.0
Ca	66900.0 ± 2400.0
Ti	2920.0 ± 330.0
Fe	29200.0 ± 1700.0
Zn	1140.0 ± 100.0
V	73.2 ± 7.0
Mn	686.0 ± 42.0
Ni	63.8 ± 3.4
Cu	104.0 ± 12.0
As	90.2 ± 10.7
Sr	469.0 ± 16.0
Cd	5.6 ± 0.4
Ba	874.0 ± 65.0
Pb	403.0 ± 32.0
U	4.3 ± 0.3

(d)

Element	Mass fraction (ppm)
Fluoranthene	7
Pyrene	4
Benz (a) anthracene	2
Benzo (b) anthracene	11
Benzo (k) anthracene	2
Benzo (a) pyrene	0.9
Benzo (a) perylene	2
Indeno (1,2,3-cd) pyrene	3

Figure 1. Physical and chemical parameters of particulate matter (PM) (certified reference material (CRM) No. 28). (**a**) Scanning electron microscopic (SEM) image, (**b**) distribution of particle size, (**c**) elemental composition as mass fractions and (**d**) polycyclic aromatic hydrocarbon composition. Except for the SEM image, the figures were delivered from the National Institute for Environmental Studies (NIES), Ibaraki, Japan, CRM No. 28 certificate.

2.2. Fucosterol: Structural Analysis

The purification procedure was assisted by a bioassay guided evaluation. The sample fractions' potential to protect macrophages against PM-stimulated inflammation and cytotoxicity was used. The chemical character was monitored via thin layer chromatography (TLC). The pure compound expressed a white colored powdered texture (Supplementary Materials, Figure S1 illustrates the purification procedure; Figure S2 depicts the GCMS analysis data for the purified compound). The molecular ion peak was observed at 412.40, and this agreed with the theoretical molecular weight of fucosterol (412.69 g mol^{-1}). Further, the fragmentation pattern and relevant fragments agreed with the library spectrum of NIST 11 (the ^{1}H and ^{13}C data, which are provided in Supplementary Materials Figure S3, were used for the structure elucidation of fucosterol). Moreover, heteronuclear single-quantum coherence spectroscopy (HSQC) and heteronuclear multiple-bond correlation (HMBC) data assisted in confirming the carbon multiplicity and that the carbon positions correlated to protons. Previously published data were referred to in the structure's elucidation [25,27].

2.3. Effect of Fucosterol (FST) against PM-Induced Cell Viability and NO Production

The protective effect of fucosterol (FST) on PM-induced macrophages are demonstrated in Figure 2. Cell viability, which was significantly affected by PM, recovered with FST exhibiting its cytoprotective effect. NO production, which was upregulated via PM, was significantly and dose-dependently downregulated through treatment with FST. LPS was used as a reference standard to compare against the data from the PM stimulation. Accordingly, LPS affected the macrophages above the level of the PM stimulation.

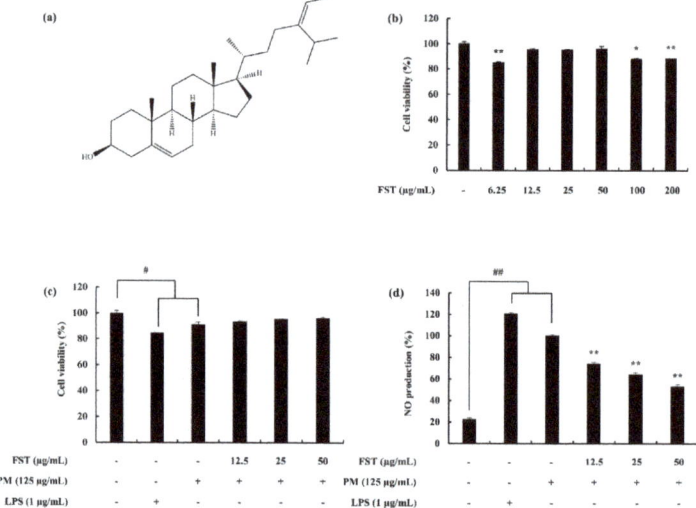

Figure 2. (a) Fucosterol (FST) skeletal formula, (b) cytotoxicity data for the FST sample against macrophages, (c) cell viability and (d) NO production of RAW macrophages against PM/LPS-stimulated conditions and the potential of FST to inhibit them. Cells were seeded and treated with FST after 24 h, incubated for 1 h and then co-treated with PM (125 µg/mL)/LPS (1 µg/mL). Triplicated experiments were used to evaluate the data. The results are represented as the mean ± SD. * $p < 0.05$, ** $p < 0.01$. # Denotes significance compared to the control, * represents significance compared to the PM treated group.

2.4. Potential of FST to Inhibit Inflammatory Mediators Driven through PM, Measured via ELISA, Western Blotting and mRNA Analysis

Pro-inflammatory cytokines (i.e., interleukin-1 (IL-1β), interleukin-6 (IL-6) and tumor necrosis factor-α (TNF-α)) lead to the upregulation of inflammatory end products. It was observed to be successfully downregulated with FST treatment (Figure 3). Prostaglandin E2 (PGE$_2$) correlated with the cyclooxygenase-2 (COX-2), while inducible nitric oxide synthase (iNOS) catalyzing the production of NO was downregulated. These results were evident through gene expression levels as well as the Western blot results (Figure 4).

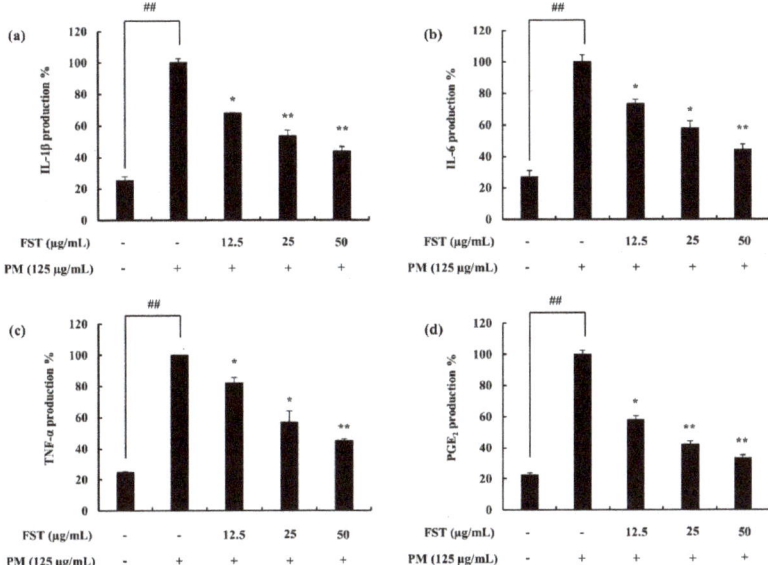

Figure 3. Assessing the pro-inflammatory cytokine inhibition activity of FST in PM-stimulated RAW 264.7 macrophages using enzyme-linked immunosorbent assay (ELISA) techniques. (**a**) Interleukin-1 (IL-1β), (**b**) interleukin-6 (IL-6), (**c**) tumor necrosis factor-α (TNF-α) and (**d**) prostaglandin E2 (PGE$_2$). Culture supernatants of RAW 264.7 cells after successive treatment of PM were used to quantify the inflammatory cytokines and PGE$_2$. Triplicated experiments were used to evaluate the data and the results are represented as the mean ± SD. * $p < 0.05$, ** $p < 0.01$. # Denotes significance compared to the control, * represents significance compared to the PM treated group.

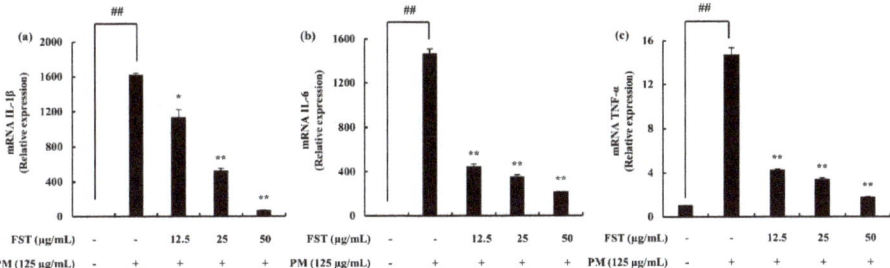

Figure 4. Cont.

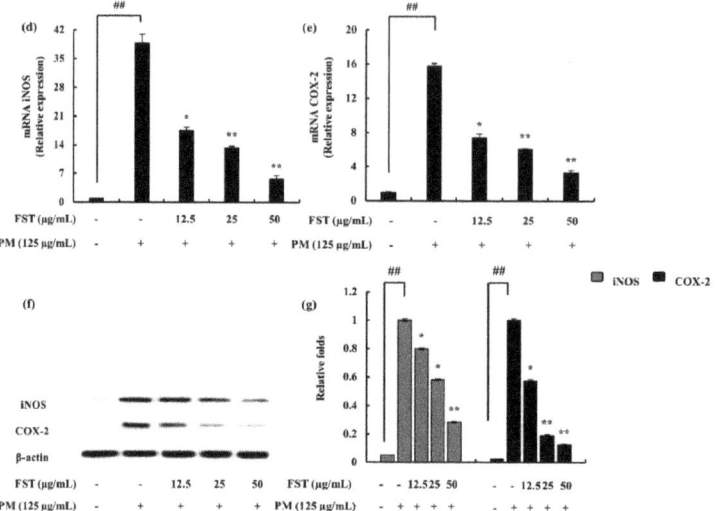

Figure 4. Gene expression analysis using RT-qPCR techniques. (**a**) IL-1β, (**b**) IL-6, (**c**) TNF-α, (**d**) inducible nitric oxide synthase (iNOS) and (**e**) cyclooxygenase-2 (COX-2). The $2^{-\Delta\Delta Ct}$ method was used to calculate the relative mRNA levels. GAPDH was used as an internal reference. Triplicated experiments were conducted. mRNA significance relative to non-treated control was calculated using the Mann–Whitney U test. * $p < 0.05$, ** $p < 0.01$. Inflammatory mediators (**f**) iNOS and COX-2 and (**g**) quantitative data were measured using Western blotting. β-actin (for cytoplasm) was used as internal control. Quantitative data was analyzed using ImageJ software. The results are expressed as the mean ± SD of three separate experiments. * $p < 0.05$, ** $p < 0.01$. # Denotes significance compared to the control while * represents significance compared to the PM-treated group.

The phosphorylation of transcription factors led to the production of inflammatory cytokines, hence, continuing the chain of inflammatory signaling. The results explain the decline in the phosphorylation of NF-κB signals, inferring the inhibition of inflammation through the particular pathway. Similarly, MAPK phosphorylation was downregulated through the activity of FST (Figure 5).

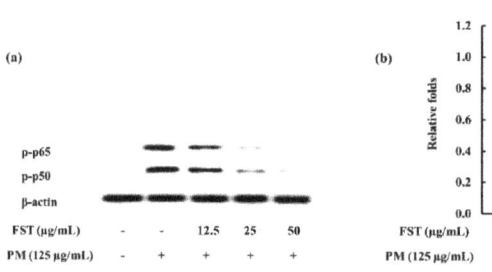
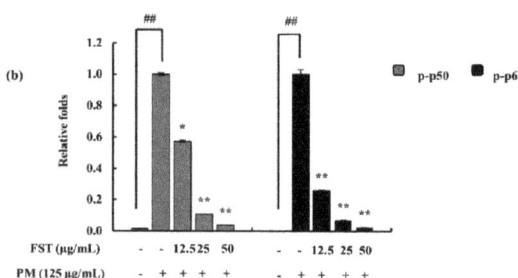

Figure 5. *Cont.*

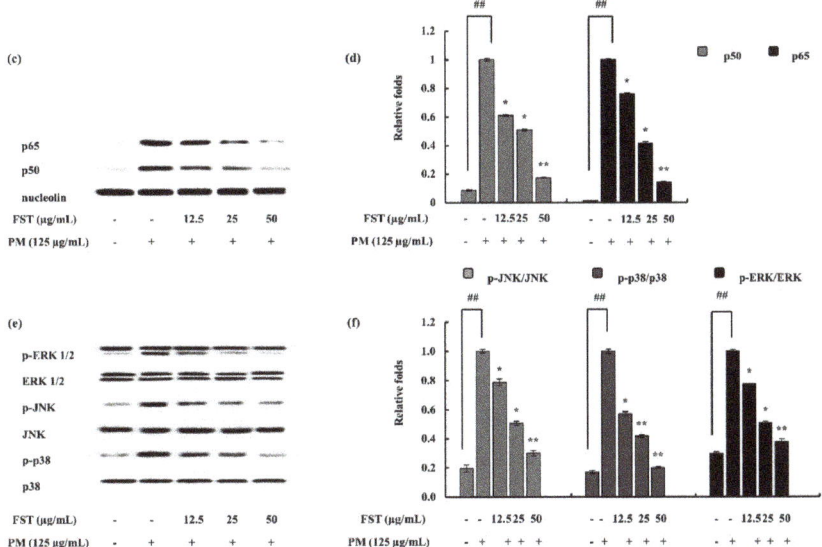

Figure 5. Evaluation of nuclear factor kappa-B (NF-κB) and mitogen-activated protein kinase (MAPK) pathway proteins in macrophages under PM-stimulated and FST-treated conditions. Data were obtained via Western blotting techniques and subsequent quantification of them with the use of ImageJ software. (**a**) p50 and p65 in cytosol, (**b**) quantitative data, (**c**) p50 and p65 in nucleus, (**d**) quantitative data, (**e**) p38, JNK and ERK and relevant (**f**) quantitative data. β-actin (for cytoplasm) and nucleolin (for nucleus) were used as internal controls. Results are expressed as the mean ± SD of three separate experiments. * $p < 0.05$, ** $p < 0.01$. # Denotes significance compared to the control while * represents significance compared to the PM-treated group.

2.5. Relation to ROS via the Oxidative Stress Pathway

The combination of the antioxidant response element (ARE) and nuclear factor erythroid 2-related factor 2 (Nrf2) plays a vital role concerning the cellular defense mechanism through the activation of a wide array of antioxidants as well as detoxification components on a transcriptional level. During dormant conditions of the cell, Nrf2 is attached with Kelch-like ECH-associated protein 1 (Keap1) in the cytoplasm; under stressful conditions, Nrf2 is dissociated from the above complex and translocated to the nucleus [28].

Western blotting was implemented to observe the expression of Nrf2 and Keap1 in the presence and absence of FST under PM-stimulated conditions. It was well observed that Nrf2 expression was upregulated under PM stimulation and, with FST, significantly activated with reference to the control. The resulting antioxidant transcription factor, HO-1, was evidently upregulated in a dose-dependent manner (Figure 6).

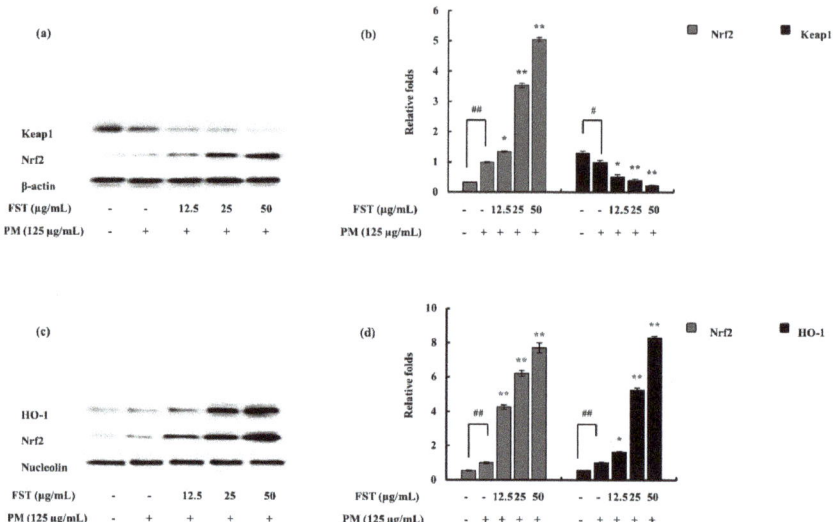

Figure 6. Effect of FST on PM-stimulated oxidative stress pathway-related proteins and their evaluation via Western blotting. (**a**) Nuclear factor erythroid 2-related factor 2 (Nrf2) and Kelch-like ECH-associated protein 1 (Keap1) in cytosol and their (**b**) quantitative data. (**c**) HO-1 and Nrf2 in the nucleus and respective (**d**) quantitative data. * $p < 0.05$, ** $p < 0.01$ versus the PM-treated group or # $p < 0.05$, ## $p < 0.01$ versus the un-stimulated group. β-actin (for cytoplasm) and nucleolin (for nucleus) were used as internal controls. Quantitative data were analyzed using ImageJ software. Results are expressed as the mean ± SD of three separate experiments. * $p < 0.05$, ** $p < 0.01$. # Denotes significance compared to the control while * represents significance compared to the PM-treated group.

3. Discussion

Air pollution can be referred to as the accumulation of diverse pollutants in the atmospheric phase of the globe, which eventually causes harm to humans and other living organisms including the natural environment [29,30]. It is reported that there is an estimated death toll above two million around the globe annually due to the direct causes of air pollution. Further, the damage is stated to effect the respiratory system [31]. The composition of PM is complex including both solid and liquid matter in varying sizes and chemical arrangements [32]. It was determined that exposure to particulate matter causes numerous health issues such as respiratory symptoms, cardiovascular diseases, lung function disputes and premature mortality [33,34].

Brown algae are widely used in the East Asia region as a food, nutraceutical and a pharmaceutical source. These include a variety of biological properties including as an antioxidant [35], anti-inflammatory [16] and antidiabetic [36]. This study selected a brown algae species, *P. boryana*, which is abundant in the Laccadive Sea, especially along the shores of Fulhadhoo Island in the Maldives. *Padina* is a calcified brown alga, and the thallus is flattened and fan shaped. The distribution of the genus is marked in temperate and tropical waters [37]. This study focused on the hexane fraction of the ethanol extract of *P. boryana*. The hexane fraction mainly contains sterols and lipids. In a majority of eukaryotic cells, sterols are present as a significant family of lipids. Sterol synthesis follows different routes and due to the fact of this reason, exhibits alterations among family classifications. Fucosterol is identified as a primary sterol in brown algae. Sanchez-Machado et al. (2004) reports that in brown seaweed fucosterol is present above 80% among sterols [38].

The results indicated a dose-dependent downregulation against PM-induced inflammation PM can easily penetrate through the respiratory tract. Human health is affected by these particles, and in due course it could result in detrimental issues, including complications in the respiratory tract and lead to allergic reactions and inflammation-caused responses in macrophage cells. As the human body consists of natural defense mechanisms, alveolar macrophages mark the first line of defense. Alveolar macrophages are involved in phagocytosis of inhaled particles. As a model system during our study, the RAW 264.7 cell line was used. Against alien challenge and tissue injury, inflammation is a constructive host defense in order to restore the structure and function of the relevant systems. Both innate and adaptive immune responses are used depending on the situation by the human body [39]. Persistent inflammation can cause non-favorable conditions such as arthritis, multiple sclerosis and inflammatory bowel disease. Anti-inflammatory agents are used in the process and act via different mechanisms. Non-steroidal anti-inflammatory drugs (NSAIDs) are frequently used as treatments, and they do not modify the pathogenesis of inflammation [40].

The cell viability which was significantly affected due to the presence of PM was successfully restored due to the treatment with FST. Inflammatory mediators, such as PGE_2, were also inhibited by the potential of FST. The ELISA evaluation of the pro-inflammatory cytokines, such as IL-6, IL-1β and TNF-α, suggested the potent activity of FST. Similarly, iNOS and COX-2 were also observed to be downregulated. Among these, iNOS is important in the production of NO, while PGE_2 production is influenced via COX-2. iNOS is one of the many isoforms in the family of nitric oxide synthases (NOSs). Similarly, COX-2 is also a member of the COX family of enzymes and primarily regulates the production of PGE_2 against inflammatory conditions [41,42].

Cytokines can be defined as proteins involved in intercellular communication. These are macromolecular proteins with higher molecular weights. Soluble cytokines are abundant while some can exist both in soluble and membrane-bound forms [43]. The cytokine level measurement was conducted using numerous methods. Two major methods implied were cytokine immunoassays using protein levels (i.e., ELISA) and mRNA levels by RT-qPCR.

The NF-κB pathway's active molecules, p50 and p65, reside in their inactive forms in the cytosol as an IκB complex. Once the stimuli is passed, the free forms of p50 and p65 translocate to the nucleus leading to the transcription of pro-inflammatory modulators [44]. The results indicate that under PM-stimulated conditions, FST downregulates phosphorylated forms in the cytosol. Nuclear p50 and p65 levels were also downregulated. The combined results suggest the potential of FST to inhibit PM-stimulated phosphorylation of the above complex, hence leading to anti-inflammatory effects. Mitogen-activated protein kinases are a family of serine/threonine protein kinases. Against external stimuli (i.e., stress signals), MAPKs support to mediate basic biological processes via regulation of the synthesis of inflammatory mediators. This makes MAPKs potential cross-points in inflammation therapeutics [45]. The activation of the MAPK pathway leads to the activation of the transcription factor NF-κB [46]. Humans possess three distinct MAP kinase cascades: extracellular signal-regulated kinases (ERK1/2), c-Jun N-terminal kinase (JNK) and p38 MAP kinase. These are activated via different MAP kinase kinases (MKKs). Among them MKK2 is responsible for the activation of ERK, while JNK is triggered via MKK 4 and 7. p38 is activated through three MKKs, namely, MKK 3, 4 and 6 [47,48]. Cell growth, differentiation besides cell death and inflammation are associated with the p38 MAP kinase pathway [49]. Earlier studies report on the potential of fucosterol to inhibit the LPS-stimulated phosphorylation of p38 MAPK and MKK 3/6. Moreover, several studies have shown the influence of p38 MAPK with regard to the activation of NF-κB [50,51]. Hence, the results of our study can be correlated with the above, such that the p38 MAPK was downregulated significantly due to the FST treatment, and the NF-κB pathway evaluation signals (i.e., p50 and p65 phosphorylation) behaved in a similar manner. However, further studies regarding MKKs are required to solidify our results in between MAPK and NF-κB.

Nrf2/HO-1, which is an evolutionary conserved mechanism, was used briefly to assess ROS involvement in the inflammatory diseases. Keap1 is an inhibitor protein, a cysteine-rich protein which is anchored to an actin cytoskeleton. It is responsible for the cytosolic sequestration of Nrf2 under physiological conditions. Keap1 promotes ubiquitination and degradation of Nrf2 under normal physiological conditions. Under stressful conditions, in which the Nrf2-dependent cellular mechanism is active (electrophiles and oxidants are rich in this stage), Nrf2 is rapidly released from Keap1. Dissociated Nrf2 is translocated to the nucleus and binds to ARE. Keap1 also receives redox information or environmental cues via its highly reactive cysteine residues, and it is referred to as the sensor of the Nrf2–Keap1 system. The dissociation of the system is a relatively rapid event. The Nrf2 half-life time is approximately 20 min [52]. The breakdown of the system leads to Keap1 stabilization. Nrf2 also increases its half-life [53]. This allows for successful nuclear translocation and cytoprotective gene transcription (HO-1) [54]. The FST treatment disrupted the Keap1/Nrf2 association while promoting its translocation to the nucleus and stabilization of Keap1 in the cytosolic environment.

The experimental results specified that the PM stimulated MAPK and NF-κB pathway mediator molecules further activating inflammatory cytokines that were significantly downregulated by FST treatment. PM air pollution has become an immense environmental and health concern not only in the East Asian region but around the globe in multiple magnitudes. Improved understanding of cellular responses related to PM stimulation would be advantageous in counteracting its detrimental effects. *P. boryana* fucosterol exhibited its effectiveness against PM-induced inflammation and related oxidative stress in RAW 264.7 macrophages as a model. The results could be utilized in the development of steroidal anti-inflammatory drugs, such as inhalers, to counteract airway inflammatory allergies. Thus, with extended in vivo scale studies, particulate matter airway complications relief can be expected.

4. Materials and Methods

4.1. Materials

China fine dust particulate matter (PM) (certified reference material No. 28) was purchased from the National Institute for Environmental Studies, Ibaraki, Japan. The organic solvents used in the experiments were of HPLC grade and were purchased from Sigma-Aldrich (St Louis, MO, USA). Silica gel 60 F254 TLC plates were purchased from Merck (Darmstadt, Germany). Silica (30–60 mesh), for open column preparation, was purchased from Sigma-Aldrich. Deuterated chloroform for NMR analysis was obtained from Cambridge Isotope Laboratories (Andover, MA, USA). The RAW 264.7 macrophage cell line was purchased from the Korean Cell Line Bank (KCLB, Seoul, Korea). Dulbecco's modified Eagle's medium (DMEM) with fetal bovine serum (FBS) and antibiotics (i.e., penicillin and streptomycin) purchased from GIBCO Inc. (Grand Island, NY, USA) were used as growth medium. 3-(4,5-Dimethylthiazol-2-yl)-2,5-diphenyltetrazolium bromide (MTT) was purchased from Sigma-Aldrich. The cytokine kits used in the experiments were purchased from eBioscience (San Diego, CA, USA), R&D Systems (Minneapolis, MN, USA), BD Opteia (San Diego, CA, USA) and Invitrogen (Carlsbad, CA, USA). Santa Cruz Biotechnology (Santa Cruz, CA, USA) purchased antibodies were used for Western blotting.

4.2. Fucosterol

4.2.1. Isolation of Fucosterol from *P. boryana*

P. boryana samples were collected from the Fulhadhoo Island coastal area of the Maldives in January 2018. Samples were immediately washed with running water to remove epiphytes and sand. The samples were then freeze-dried and powdered. Sample repositories were stored in the Marine Bio Resource Technology Lab, Jeju National University. Sample extraction was conducted successfully with 70% ethanol four times. This was evaporated to obtain the crude ethanolic extract of *P. boryana* (PBE). PBE was dissolved in deionized water and a stepwise fractionation was conducted (hexane, chloroform and ethyl acetate). The hexane fraction was further resolved (PBEH1–PBEH5). The elution solvent consisted of hexane and ethyl acetate in increasing polarity (9:1→7:3→1:1)→ethyl acetate and ethyl acetate:methanol (1:1). A second silica open column was used to resolve the fraction PBEH2. The elution was done in the same solvent system with increasing polarity (85:15→65:35→1:1 and ethyl acetate). This resulted in four fractions (PBEH21–PBEH24). The PBEH22 was resolved, resulting a collection of 96 tubes. This was analyzed by TLC, and the tubes were pooled into four fractions (F1–F4). Fraction F2 was resolved via preparative TLC resulting in 7 fractions (F2A–F2G). Among these fractions, F2F indicated the presence of fucosterol (FST) and was identified as the active metabolite (Supplementary Materials Figure S1 details the purification and isolation procedures.) The sample was used for cell culture bioassays after dissolving in DMSO and successful serial dilution in culture media. The sample DMSO concentrations in working samples were maintained at less than 0.1% [25].

4.2.2. Structural Characterization

GC-MS assisted in the structural confirmation (Shimadzu GCMS-TQ8040, Shimadzu Corp., Kyoto, Japan). The method involved a fused silica capillary column (RTx-5MS, 30 m × 0.25 mm i.d., 0.25 µm film thickness), an injection temperature of 280 °C and was injected via splitless mode. The oven program was 260 °C, 3 min, 6 °C/min to 320 °C, 5 °C/min to 330 °C, 2 min. The ion source temperature was maintained at 200 °C. The scan range was 50–500 m/z. Helium was used as the carrier gas with a constant flow rate of 0.73 mL/min [55].

Nuclear magnetic resonance spectroscopy (NMR) was conducted using a 400 MHz spectrometer (JNM-ECX400, JEOL, Japan). ^{1}H and ^{13}C NMR spectra were successfully obtained. The sample was prepared by dissolving a minute amount in $CDCl_3$. The chemical shifts were demonstrated in ppm and the coupling constants in Hz. Multiplicity abbreviations were used as the following: s = singlet, d = doublet, t = triplet, dt = doublet of triplet, dd = doublet of doublet and m = multiplet. Heteronuclear single-quantum coherence (HSQC) and heteronuclear multiple-bond correlation (HMBC) were conducted to confirm the carbon multiplicity and carbon positions correlated to protons [25,27].

4.3. Particulate Matter: Morphological Analysis

The sample was platinum sputter coated (Quorum Technologies, Lewes, UK). The surface morphology of the CRM No. 28 particles was observed using a JSM-6700F field-emission scanning electron microscope (JEOL, Tokyo, Japan). The instrument was operated at 10.0 kV.

4.4. Cell Culture

4.4.1. Maintenance of Cell Line

The RAW 264.7 macrophage cell line was maintained in the DMEM growth medium (10% FBS and 1% antibiotics). The cells were maintained under controlled conditions: 5% CO_2 and 37 °C. Cells were periodically sub-cultured and used for experiments in the exponential growth phase.

4.4.2. Measurement of Cell Viability

Initially, the optimum FST concentration values were determined via screening a wide range. This was followed by the evaluation of the cytoprotective effect of FST against PM/LPS-stimulated macrophages. The cells were seeded with a cell concentration of 1×10^5 cells/mL (96 well plates). FST was treated after a 24 h incubation period. PM (125 µg/mL)/LPS (1 µg/mL) was treated after 1 h and continued its incubation further for 23 h. An MTT assay was performed [56]. The assay results were obtained in the 540 nm optical density value.

4.4.3. Evaluation of NO Inhibition Activity

The macrophage cell line was seeded in 24 well plates. The samples were treated and were incubated for 1 h and then stimulated with PM (125 µg/mL)/LPS (1 µg/mL). At 23 h, further incubation was continued. NO production analysis was conducted using the Griess assay [57,58].

4.5. Assessing PGE$_2$ and pro-Inflammatory Cytokine Production

Initially, the cells were seeded (24 well plates), and within 24 h the FST sample was treated. The PM (125 µg/mL) stimulation was conducted after 1 h and further incubated for 23 h. The cell media were retrieved individually and assessed for each parameter of cytokine. The manufacturer's instructions were followed in the process.

4.6. FST Downregulated NF-κB and MAPK Pathway Proteins

Inflammatory mediators, such as iNOS and COX-2, including the NF-κB pathway (i.e., p50 and p65) and MAPKs (i.e., p38, ERK and JNK), were assessed via Western blotting. Further, selected oxidative stress pathway proteins were also evaluated (i.e., Nrf2, Keap1 and HO-1). Cells were seeded (six well plates) and treated with samples and induced with PM. The cells were harvested, lysed and the proteins were measured using the BCA protein assay method. The harvesting time was dependent on the type of protein analysis and followed the method explained by Jayawardena et al. (2019) [42]. Proteins were subjected to electrophoresis (sodium sulfate–polyacrylamide gels, 12%), transferred to nitrocellulose membranes and blocked with skimmed milk. Primary and secondary antibody incubation was conducted, and the bands were ultimately developed and photographed (FUSION Solo Vilber Lourmat system). The ImageJ program was used for the band intensity quantification process [58,59].

4.7. Gene Expression Analysis

4.7.1. Extraction of RNA and cDNA Synthesis

The total RNA from the cells were extracted via a commercial extraction kit following the manufacturer's instructions (Tri-Reagent™, Sigma-Aldrich, St. Louis, MO, USA). Depending on the quantified RNA content measured (µDrop Plate, Thermo Scientific, Waltham, MA, USA), first strand cDNA was synthesized and stored at −80 °C (prime Script™, Takara Bio Inc., Kusatsu, Shiga, Japan).

4.7.2. Quantitative Real-Time PCR (qPCR) Analysis

SYBR green quantitative real-time PCR techniques were implemented to measure gene expression levels. A Thermal Cycler Dice-Real Time System (Takara, Japan) was used to complete the process. GAPDH was the internal reference standard. The experimental method followed the process explained by Jayawardena et al. (2019) [42]. Data were analyzed using the method explained by Livak and Schmittgen (2001) [60].

GAPDH, antisense; 5'-AAGGGTCATCATCTCTGCCC-3' and sense, 5'-GTGATGGCATGGACTGTGGT -3';
IL-1β, antisense; 5'-CAGGATGAGGACATGAGCACC-3' and sense, 5'-CTCTGCAGACTCAAACTCCAC -3';
IL-6, antisense; 5'-GTACTCCAGAAGACCAGAGG -3' and sense, 5'-TGCTGGTGACAACCACGGCC-3';
TNF-α, antisense; 5'-TTGACCTCAGCGCTGAGTTG -3' and sense, 5'-CCTGTAGCCCACGTCGTAGC -3';
iNOS, antisense; 5'-ATGTCCGAAGCAAACATCAC-3' and sense, 5'-TAATGTCCAGGAAGTAGGTG-3';
COX2, antisense; 5'-CAGCAAATCCTTGCTGTTCC -3' and sense, 5'-TGGGCAAAGAATGCAAACATC-3'.

4.8. Statistical Analysis

The experiments were conducted in triplicate and data are expressed as the mean ± standard deviation. Data were analyzed using IBM SPSS with one-way ANOVA. * $p < 0.05$, * $p < 0.01$ versus the PM-treated group or $^{\#}\,p < 0.05$, $^{\#\#}\,p < 0.01$ versus the un-stimulated group were considered statistically significant.

5. Conclusions

Fucosterol purified from *P. boryana* exhibited an effective potential against PM-induced inflammatory conditions in RAW 264.7 macrophages. NO, the distinct end product of inflammation, was successfully inhibited via fucosterol under PM-stimulated conditions. Inflammatory mediators, such as iNOS, COX-2 and PGE$_2$ as well as pro-inflammatory cytokines (i.e., IL-1β, IL-6 and TNF-α), were observed to be downregulated dose-dependently with the treatment of FST. These results were further reinforced via the MAPK and NF-κB pathway signal molecule expression subdual. The Nrf2/HO-1 pathway results suggest ROS downregulation due to the activity of fucosterol. Thus, fucosterol could function as a potent protector against PM-induced inflammatory diseases. In conclusion, this study provides an understanding of PM-stimulated cellular responses and mechanisms. Further, in vivo studies would be beneficial to understand the detailed mechanisms and bioavailability of fucosterol on target organs.

Supplementary Materials: The following are available online at http://www.mdpi.com/1660-3397/18/12/628/s1, Figure S1. Flow diagram representing the extraction and fractionation of *Padina boryana* (PC) 70% ethanol extract (PBE). Figure S2. GC-MS/MS analysis of fucosterol. Figure S3. ^{1}H and ^{13}C NMR spectrum of fucosterol.

Author Contributions: Conceptualization, Y.-J.J. and T.U.J.; methodology, T.U.J.; software, D.P.N., H.-W.Y., H.-G.L.; validation, T.U.J., K.K.A.S.; formal analysis, T.U.J.; investigation, T.U.J.; resources, D.P.N., H.-G.L., H.-W.Y.; data curation, M.-C.K.; writing—original draft preparation, T.U.J.; writing—review and editing, T.U.J. and Y.-J.J.; supervision, Y.-J.J.; project administration, Y.-J.J.; funding acquisition, Y.-J.J. All authors have read and agreed to the published version of the manuscript.

Funding: This research was financially supported by a grant from the "Marine Biotechnology program—20170488", funded by the Ministry of Oceans and Fisheries, Korea.

Conflicts of Interest: The authors declare to possess no competing interests.

References

1. Lin, Z.-C.; Lee, C.-W.; Tsai, M.-H.; Ko, H.-H.; Fang, J.-Y.; Chiang, Y.-C.; Liang, C.-J.; Hsu, L.-F.; Hu, S.C.-S.; Yen, F.-L. Eupafolin nanoparticles protect HaCaT keratinocytes from particulate matter-induced inflammation and oxidative stress. *Int. J. Nanomed.* **2016**, *11*, 3907–3926. [CrossRef]
2. Wang, W.; Primbs, T.; Tao, S.; Simonich, S.L. Atmospheric particulate matter pollution during the 2008 Beijing Olympics. *Environ. Sci. Technol.* **2009**, *43*, 5314–5320. [CrossRef] [PubMed]
3. Lee, Y.G.; Ho, C.H.; Kim, J.H.; Kim, J. Quiescence of Asian dust events in South Korea and Japan during 2012 spring: Dust outbreaks and transports. *Atmos. Environ.* **2015**, *114*, 92–101. [CrossRef]
4. Maxwell-Meier, K. Inorganic composition of fine particles in mixed mineral dust–pollution plumes observed from airborne measurements during ACE-Asia. *J. Geophys. Res.* **2004**, *109*. [CrossRef]
5. Harrison, R.M.; Yin, J. Particulate matter in the atmosphere: Which particle properties are important for its effects on health? *Sci. Total Environ.* **2000**, *249*, 85–101. [CrossRef]
6. Lv, B.L.; Zhang, B.; Bai, Y.Q. A systematic analysis of PM2.5 in Beijing and its sources from 2000 to 2012. *Atmos. Environ.* **2016**, *124*, 98–108. [CrossRef]
7. Wall, S.M.; John, W.; Ondo, J.L. Measurement of Aerosol Size Distributions for Nitrate and Major Ionic Species. *Atmos. Environ.* **1988**, *22*, 1649–1656. [CrossRef]
8. Dreher, K.; Jaskot, R.; Kodavanti, U.; Lehmann, J.; Winsett, D.; Costa, D. Soluble transition metals mediate the acute pulmonary injury and airway hyperreactivity induced by residual oil fly ash particles. *Chest* **1996**, *109*, 33S–34S. [CrossRef]
9. Kodavanti, U.P.; Jaskot, R.H.; Su, W.Y.; Costa, D.L.; Ghio, A.J.; Dreher, K.L. Genetic variability in combustion particle-induced chronic lung injury. *Am. J. Physiol.* **1997**, *272*, L521–L532. [CrossRef]
10. Becker, S.; Soukup, J.M.; Gilmour, M.I.; Devlin, R.B. Stimulation of human and rat alveolar macrophages by urban air particulates: Effects on oxidant radical generation and cytokine production. *Toxicol. Appl. Pharmacol.* **1996**, *141*, 637–648. [CrossRef] [PubMed]

11. Pritchard, R.J.; Ghio, A.J.; Lehmann, J.R.; Winsett, D.W.; Tepper, J.S.; Park, P.; Gilmour, M.I.; Dreher, K.L.; Costa, D.L. Oxidant generation and lung injury after particulate air pollutant exposure increase with the concentrations of associated metals. *Inhal. Toxicol.* **1996**, *8*, 457–477. [CrossRef]
12. Shukla, A.; Timblin, C.; BeruBe, K.; Gordon, T.; McKinney, W.; Driscoll, K.; Vacek, P.; Mossman, B.T. Inhaled particulate matter causes expression of nuclear factor (NF)-kappaB-related genes and oxidant-dependent NF-kappaB activation in vitro. *Am. J. Respir. Cell Mol. Biol.* **2000**, *23*, 182–187. [CrossRef] [PubMed]
13. Zhao, Q.; Chen, H.; Yang, T.; Rui, W.; Liu, F.; Zhang, F.; Zhao, Y.; Ding, W. Direct effects of airborne PM2.5 exposure on macrophage polarizations. *Biochim. Biophys. Acta* **2016**, *1860*, 2835–2843. [CrossRef] [PubMed]
14. Cho, Y.S.; Moon, H.B. The role of oxidative stress in the pathogenesis of asthma. *Allergy Asthma Immunol. Res.* **2010**, *2*, 183–187. [CrossRef]
15. Bernard, K.; Hecker, L.; Luckhardt, T.R.; Cheng, G.; Thannickal, V.J. NADPH oxidases in lung health and disease. *Antioxid. Redox Signal.* **2014**, *20*, 2838–2853. [CrossRef]
16. Heo, S.J.; Yoon, W.J.; Kim, K.N.; Ahn, G.N.; Kang, S.M.; Kang, D.H.; Affan, A.; Oh, C.; Jung, W.K.; Jeon, Y.J. Evaluation of anti-inflammatory effect of fucoxanthin isolated from brown algae in lipopolysaccharide-stimulated RAW 264.7 macrophages. *Food Chem. Toxicol.* **2010**, *48*, 2045–2051. [CrossRef]
17. Jang, K.H.; Lee, B.H.; Choi, B.W.; Lee, H.S.; Shin, J. Chromenes from the brown alga *Sargassum siliquastrum*. *J. Nat. Prod.* **2005**, *68*, 716–723. [CrossRef]
18. Heo, S.J.; Kim, J.P.; Jung, W.K.; Lee, N.H.; Kang, H.S.; Jun, E.M.; Park, S.H.; Kang, S.M.; Lee, Y.J.; Park, P.J.; et al. Identification of chemical structure and free radical scavenging activity of diphlorethohydroxycarmalol isolated from a brown alga, *Ishige okamurae*. *J. Microbiol. Biotechnol.* **2008**, *18*, 676–681.
19. Shanura Fernando, I.P.; Asanka Sanjeewa, K.K.; Samarakoon, K.W.; Lee, W.W.; Kim, H.S.; Ranasinghe, P.; Gunasekara, U.; Jeon, Y.J. Antioxidant and anti-inflammatory functionality of ten Sri Lankan seaweed extracts obtained by carbohydrase assisted extraction. *Food Sci. Biotechnol.* **2018**, *27*, 1761–1769. [CrossRef]
20. Usoltseva, R.V.; Anastyuk, S.D.; Ishina, I.A.; Isakov, V.V.; Zvyagintseva, T.N.; Thinh, P.D.; Zadorozhny, P.A.; Dmitrenok, P.S.; Ermakova, S.P. Structural characteristics and anticancer activity in vitro of fucoidan from brown alga *Padina boryana*. *Carbohydr. Polym.* **2018**, *184*, 260–268. [CrossRef]
21. Heilbron, I.; Phipers, R.F.; Wright, H.R. 343. The chemistry of the algæ. Part I. The algal sterol fucosterol. *J. Chem. Soc.* **1934**, 1572–1576. [CrossRef]
22. Lee, S.; Lee, Y.S.; Jung, S.H.; Kang, S.S.; Shin, K.H. Anti-oxidant activities of fucosterol from the marine algae *Pelvetia siliquosa*. *Arch. Pharm. Res.* **2003**, *26*, 719–722. [CrossRef] [PubMed]
23. Jung, H.A.; Jin, S.E.; Ahn, B.R.; Lee, C.M.; Choi, J.S. Anti-inflammatory activity of edible brown alga *Eisenia bicyclis* and its constituents fucosterol and phlorotannins in LPS-stimulated RAW264.7 macrophages. *Food Chem. Toxicol.* **2013**, *59*, 199–206. [CrossRef] [PubMed]
24. Bang, M.H.; Kim, H.H.; Lee, D.Y.; Han, M.W.; Baek, Y.S.; Chung, D.K.; Baek, N.I. Anti-osteoporotic activities of fucosterol from sea mustard (*Undaria pinnatifida*). *Food Sci. Biotechnol.* **2011**, *20*, 343–347. [CrossRef]
25. Fernando, I.P.S.; Jayawardena, T.U.; Kim, H.S.; Lee, W.W.; Vaas, A.; De Silva, H.I.C.; Abayaweera, G.S.; Nanayakkara, C.M.; Abeytunga, D.T.U.; Lee, D.S.; et al. Beijing urban particulate matter-induced injury and inflammation in human lung epithelial cells and the protective effects of fucosterol from *Sargassum binderi* (Sonder ex J. Agardh). *Environ. Res.* **2019**, *172*, 150–158. [CrossRef] [PubMed]
26. Mori, I.; Sun, Z.; Ukachi, M.; Nagano, K.; McLeod, C.W.; Cox, A.G.; Nishikawa, M. Development and certification of the new NIES CRM 28: Urban aerosols for the determination of multielements. *Anal. Bioanal. Chem.* **2008**, *391*, 1997–2003. [CrossRef] [PubMed]
27. Suttiarporn, P.; Chumpolsri, W.; Mahatheeranont, S.; Luangkamin, S.; Teepsawang, S.; Leardkamolkarn, V. Structures of phytosterols and triterpenoids with potential anti-cancer activity in bran of black non-glutinous rice. *Nutrients* **2015**, *7*, 1672–1687. [CrossRef]
28. Gasparrini, M.; Afrin, S.; Forbes-Hernandez, T.Y.; Cianciosi, D.; Reboredo-Rodriguez, P.; Amici, A.; Battino, M.; Giampieri, F. Protective effects of Manuka honey on LPS-treated RAW 264.7 macrophages. Part 2: Control of oxidative stress induced damage, increase of antioxidant enzyme activities and attenuation of inflammation. *Food Chem. Toxicol.* **2018**, *120*, 578–587. [CrossRef]
29. Kinney, P.L. Climate change, air quality, and human health. *Am. J. Prev. Med.* **2008**, *35*, 459–467. [CrossRef]
30. Brauer, M.; Amann, M.; Burnett, R.T.; Cohen, A.; Dentener, F.; Ezzati, M.; Henderson, S.B.; Krzyzanowski, M.; Martin, R.V.; Van Dingenen, R.; et al. Exposure assessment for estimation of the global burden of disease attributable to outdoor air pollution. *Environ. Sci. Technol.* **2012**, *46*, 652–660. [CrossRef]

31. Shah, A.S.; Langrish, J.P.; Nair, H.; McAllister, D.A.; Hunter, A.L.; Donaldson, K.; Newby, D.E.; Mills, N.L. Global association of air pollution and heart failure: A systematic review and meta-analysis. *Lancet* **2013**, *382*, 1039–1048. [CrossRef]
32. Kim, K.H.; Kabir, E.; Kabir, S. A review on the human health impact of airborne particulate matter. *Environ. Int.* **2015**, *74*, 136–143. [CrossRef]
33. Guaita, R.; Pichiule, M.; Mate, T.; Linares, C.; Diaz, J. Short-term impact of particulate matter (PM(2.5)) on respiratory mortality in Madrid. *Int. J. Environ. Health Res.* **2011**, *21*, 260–274. [CrossRef] [PubMed]
34. Perez, L.; Tobias, A.; Querol, X.; Pey, J.; Alastuey, A.; Diaz, J.; Sunyer, J. Saharan dust, particulate matter and cause-specific mortality: A case-crossover study in Barcelona (Spain). *Environ. Int.* **2012**, *48*, 150–155. [CrossRef] [PubMed]
35. Heo, S.J.; Park, E.J.; Lee, K.W.; Jeon, Y.J. Antioxidant activities of enzymatic extracts from brown seaweeds. *Bioresour. Technol.* **2005**, *96*, 1613–1623. [CrossRef]
36. Lee, S.H.; Jeon, Y.J. Anti-diabetic effects of brown algae derived phlorotannins, marine polyphenols through diverse mechanisms. *Fitoterapia* **2013**, *86*, 129–136. [CrossRef]
37. Hanyuda, T.; Arai, S.; Uchimura, M.; Abbott, I.A.; Kawai, H. Three new records of Padina in Japan based on morphological and molecular markers. *Phycol. Res.* **2008**, *56*, 288–300. [CrossRef]
38. Sanchez-Machado, D.I.; Lopez-Hernandez, J.; Paseiro-Losada, P.; Lopez-Cervantes, J. An HPLC method for the quantification of sterols in edible seaweeds. *Biomed. Chromatogr.* **2004**, *18*, 183–190. [CrossRef]
39. Lawrence, T.; Willoughby, D.A.; Gilroy, D.W. Anti-inflammatory lipid mediators and insights into the resolution of inflammation. *Nat. Rev. Immunol.* **2002**, *2*, 787–795. [CrossRef]
40. Abdul, Q.A.; Choi, R.J.; Jung, H.A.; Choi, J.S. Health benefit of fucosterol from marine algae: A review. *J. Sci. Food Agric.* **2016**, *96*, 1856–1866. [CrossRef]
41. Alderton, W.K.; Cooper, C.E.; Knowles, R.G. Nitric oxide synthases: Structure, function and inhibition. *Biochem. J.* **2001**, *357*, 593–615. [CrossRef] [PubMed]
42. Jayawardena, T.U.; Kim, H.-S.; Sanjeewa, K.K.A.; Kim, S.-Y.; Rho, J.-R.; Jee, Y.; Ahn, G.; Jeon, Y.-J. *Sargassum horneri* and isolated 6-hydroxy-4,4,7a-trimethyl-5,6,7,7a-tetrahydrobenzofuran-2(4H)-one (HTT); LPS-induced inflammation attenuation via suppressing NF-κB, MAPK and oxidative stress through Nrf2/HO-1 pathways in RAW 264.7 macrophages. *Algal Res.* **2019**, *40*, 101513. [CrossRef]
43. Nicola, N. *Guidebook to Cytokines and Their Receptors*; Oxford University Press: Oxford, UK, 1994.
44. Li, Q.; Verma, I.M. NF-kappaB regulation in the immune system. *Nat. Rev. Immunol.* **2002**, *2*, 725–734. [CrossRef] [PubMed]
45. Kaminska, B. MAPK signalling pathways as molecular targets for anti-inflammatory therapy—From molecular mechanisms to therapeutic benefits. *Biochim. Biophys. Acta* **2005**, *1754*, 253–262. [CrossRef]
46. Tak, P.P.; Firestein, G.S. NF-kappaB: A key role in inflammatory diseases. *J. Clin. Investig.* **2001**, *107*, 7–11. [CrossRef] [PubMed]
47. Pearson, G.; Robinson, F.; Beers Gibson, T.; Xu, B.E.; Karandikar, M.; Berman, K.; Cobb, M.H. Mitogen-activated protein (MAP) kinase pathways: Regulation and physiological functions. *Endocr. Rev.* **2001**, *22*, 153–183. [CrossRef]
48. Raingeaud, J.; Whitmarsh, A.J.; Barrett, T.; Derijard, B.; Davis, R.J. MKK3- and MKK6-regulated gene expression is mediated by the p38 mitogen-activated protein kinase signal transduction pathway. *Mol. Cell. Biol.* **1996**, *16*, 1247–1255. [CrossRef]
49. Kyriakis, J.M.; Avruch, J. Mammalian mitogen-activated protein kinase signal transduction pathways activated by stress and inflammation. *Physiol. Rev.* **2001**, *81*, 807–869. [CrossRef]
50. Yoo, M.S.; Shin, J.S.; Choi, H.E.; Cho, Y.W.; Bang, M.H.; Baek, N.I.; Lee, K.T. Fucosterol isolated from *Undaria pinnatifida* inhibits lipopolysaccharide-induced production of nitric oxide and pro-inflammatory cytokines via the inactivation of nuclear factor-kappaB and p38 mitogen-activated protein kinase in RAW264.7 macrophages. *Food Chem.* **2012**, *135*, 967–975. [CrossRef]
51. Rao, K.M.; Meighan, T.; Bowman, L. Role of mitogen-activated protein kinase activation in the production of inflammatory mediators: Differences between primary rat alveolar macrophages and macrophage cell lines. *J. Toxicol. Environ. Health A* **2002**, *65*, 757–768. [CrossRef]

52. Kobayashi, M.; Li, L.; Iwamoto, N.; Nakajima-Takagi, Y.; Kaneko, H.; Nakayama, Y.; Eguchi, M.; Wada, Y.; Kumagai, Y.; Yamamoto, M. The antioxidant defense system Keap1-Nrf2 comprises a multiple sensing mechanism for responding to a wide range of chemical compounds. *Mol. Cell. Biol.* **2009**, *29*, 493–502. [CrossRef] [PubMed]
53. Canning, P.; Sorrell, F.J.; Bullock, A.N. Structural basis of Keap1 interactions with Nrf2. *Free Radic. Biol. Med.* **2015**, *88*, 101–107. [CrossRef] [PubMed]
54. Loboda, A.; Jazwa, A.; Grochot-Przeczek, A.; Rutkowski, A.J.; Cisowski, J.; Agarwal, A.; Jozkowicz, A.; Dulak, J. Heme oxygenase-1 and the vascular bed: From molecular mechanisms to therapeutic opportunities. *Antioxid. Redox Signal.* **2008**, *10*, 1767–1812. [CrossRef] [PubMed]
55. Fernando, I.P.S.; Lee, W.W.; Jayawardena, T.U.; Kang, M.-C.; Ann, Y.-S.; Ko, C.-I.; Park, Y.J.; Jeon, Y.-J. 3β-Hydroxy-Δ5-steroidal congeners from a column fraction of Dendronephthya puetteri attenuate LPS-induced inflammatory responses in RAW 264.7 macrophages and zebrafish embryo model. *RSC Adv.* **2018**, *8*, 18626–18634. [CrossRef]
56. Mosmann, T. Rapid colorimetric assay for cellular growth and survival: Application to proliferation and cytotoxicity assays. *J. Immunol. Methods* **1983**, *65*, 55–63. [CrossRef]
57. Wijesinghe, W.A.J.P.; Kang, M.C.; Lee, W.W.; Lee, H.S.; Kamada, T.; Vairappan, C.S.; Jeon, Y.J. 5 beta-Hydroxypalisadin B isolated from red alga *Laurencia snackeyi* attenuates inflammatory response in lipopolysaccharide-stimulated RAW 264.7 macrophages. *Algae* **2014**, *29*, 333–341. [CrossRef]
58. Jayawardena, T.U.; Asanka Sanjeewa, K.K.; Shanura Fernando, I.P.; Ryu, B.M.; Kang, M.C.; Jee, Y.; Lee, W.W.; Jeon, Y.J. *Sargassum horneri* (Turner) C. Agardh ethanol extract inhibits the fine dust inflammation response via activating Nrf2/HO-1 signaling in RAW 264.7 cells. *BMC Complement. Altern. Med.* **2018**, *18*, 249. [CrossRef]
59. Sanjeewa, K.K.A.; Jayawardena, T.U.; Kim, H.-S.; Kim, S.-Y.; Ahn, G.; Kim, H.-J.; Fu, X.; Jee, Y.; Jeon, Y.-J. Ethanol extract separated from *Sargassum horneri* (Turner) abate LPS-induced inflammation in RAW 264.7 macrophages. *Fish. Aquat. Sci.* **2019**, *22*, 6. [CrossRef]
60. Livak, K.J.; Schmittgen, T.D. Analysis of relative gene expression data using real-time quantitative PCR and the 2(-Delta Delta C(T)) Method. *Methods* **2001**, *25*, 402–408. [CrossRef]

Publisher's Note: MDPI stays neutral with regard to jurisdictional claims in published maps and institutional affiliations.

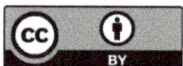

© 2020 by the authors. Licensee MDPI, Basel, Switzerland. This article is an open access article distributed under the terms and conditions of the Creative Commons Attribution (CC BY) license (http://creativecommons.org/licenses/by/4.0/).

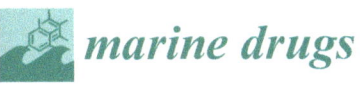

Article

Efficacy of *Posidonia oceanica* Extract against Inflammatory Pain: In Vivo Studies in Mice

Laura Micheli [1,†], Marzia Vasarri [2,†], Emanuela Barletta [2], Elena Lucarini [1], Carla Ghelardini [1], Donatella Degl'Innocenti [2,3] and Lorenzo Di Cesare Mannelli [1,*]

1. Department of Neuroscience, Psychology, Drug Research and Child Health (NEUROFARBA)-Pharmacology and Toxicology Section, University of Florence, Viale Gaetano Pieraccini, 6, 50139 Florence, Italy; laura.micheli@unifi.it (L.M.); elena.lucarini@unifi.it (E.L.); carla.ghelardini@unifi.it (C.G.)
2. Department of Experimental and Clinical Biomedical Sciences, University of Florence, Viale Morgagni 50, 50134 Florence, Italy; marzia.vasarri@unifi.it (M.V.); emanuela.barletta@unifi.it (E.B.); donatella.deglinnocenti@unifi.it (D.D.)
3. Interuniversity Center of Marine Biology and Applied Ecology "G. Bacci" (CIBM), Viale N. Sauro 4, 57128 Livorno, Italy
* Correspondence: lorenzo.mannelli@unifi.it
† These authors contribute equally to this work.

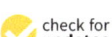

Citation: Micheli, L.; Vasarri, M.; Barletta, E.; Lucarini, E.; Ghelardini, C.; Degl'Innocenti, D.; Di Cesare Mannelli, L. Efficacy of *Posidonia oceanica* Extract against Inflammatory Pain: In Vivo Studies in Mice. *Mar. Drugs* **2021**, *19*, 48. https://doi.org/10.3390/md19020048

Received: 29 December 2020
Accepted: 19 January 2021
Published: 21 January 2021

Publisher's Note: MDPI stays neutral with regard to jurisdictional claims in published maps and institutional affiliations.

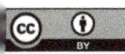

Copyright: © 2021 by the authors. Licensee MDPI, Basel, Switzerland. This article is an open access article distributed under the terms and conditions of the Creative Commons Attribution (CC BY) license (https://creativecommons.org/licenses/by/4.0/).

Abstract: *Posidonia oceanica* (L.) Delile is traditionally used for its beneficial properties. Recently, promising antioxidant and anti-inflammatory biological properties emerged through studying the in vitro activity of the ethanolic leaves extract (POE). The present study aims to investigate the anti-inflammatory and analgesic role of POE in mice. Inflammatory pain was modeled in CD-1 mice by the intraplantar injection of carrageenan, interleukin IL-1β and formalin. Pain threshold was measured by von Frey and paw pressure tests. Nociceptive pain was studied by the hot-plate test. POE (10–100 mg kg^{-1}) was administered per os. The paw soft tissue of carrageenan-treated animals was analyzed to measure anti-inflammatory and antioxidant effects. POE exerted a dose-dependent, acute anti-inflammatory effect able to counteract carrageenan-induced pain and paw oedema. Similar anti-hyperalgesic and anti-allodynic results were obtained when inflammation was induced by IL-1β. In the formalin test, the pre-treatment with POE significantly reduced the nocifensive behavior. Moreover, POE was able to evoke an analgesic effect in naïve animals. Ex vivo, POE reduced the myeloperoxidase activity as well as TNF-α and IL-1β levels; further antioxidant properties were highlighted as a reduction in NO concentration. POE is the candidate for a new valid strategy against inflammation and pain.

Keywords: *P. oceanica*; inflammation; pain; CD-1 mice

1. Introduction

Posidonia oceanica (L.) Delile is a marine vascular plant belonging to the Posidoniaceae family and the only endemic species of the Mediterranean Sea. It is a seagrass that blooms underwater forming vast meadows of tens of thousands of square kilometers of great ecological importance and is essential for the entire marine ecosystem [1].

According to tradition, *P. oceanica* provided benefits for human health. The first information on the *P. oceanica* healing properties comes from ancient Egypt, where it was assumed to be effective against sore throats and skin problems [2]. Other documents describe its traditional use to treat inflammation and irritation, but also acne, lower limbs pain and colitis [3].

A more recent tradition of the villagers of the west Anatolian coast concerns the use of *P. oceanica* leaves decoction as a natural remedy for diabetes and hypertension [4]. An in vivo preclinical study claimed that oral administration of an ethanolic extract from *P. oceanica* leaves in alloxan-induced diabetic rats lowered blood sugar, restored antioxidant enzyme activity and reduced the lipid peroxidation process, supporting the antidiabetic and vasoprotective roles of *P. oceanica* [4].

Recently, the hydroalcoholic extract from *P. oceanica* leaves, called POE, has been the focus of a series of bioactivity studies. A first UPLC characterization analysis, conducted by some of our authors [5], showed that the hydrophilic fraction of POE consisted of 88% phenolic compounds. The polyphenolic profile was specifically represented by about 85% (+) catechins, while the remaining 5% by a mixture of gallic acid (0.4%), ferulic acid (1.7%), epicatechin (1.4%) and chlorogenic acid (0.6%). The small remaining fraction (11%) was represented by minor peaks, indicating the presence of further compounds, which, although detectable as phenols, are un-known/uncharacterized (Figure 1) [5].

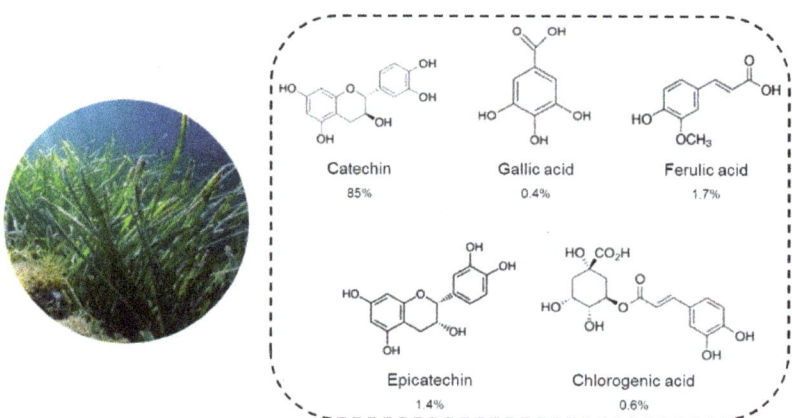

Figure 1. Phenolic profile of *P. oceanica* leaves extract (POE) obtained by UPLC analysis [5]. The percentage composition of each phenolic compound in POE is reported below each chemical structure. An additional 11% of POE composition remains unknown and/or uncharacterized.

Although the individual phenolic compounds identified have been tested in some experimental models of in vitro bioactivity [5], POE has been shown to be particularly effective as a phytocomplex. Indeed, POE has proved to be capable of inhibiting the migration of cancer cells, such as human fibrosarcoma HT1080 cells [5,6] and human neuroblastoma SH-SY5Y cells [7]. The total absence of cellular toxicity in POE activities has been attributed to its ability to modulate the activation of the autophagic process [6].

In relation to the traditional and recognized antidiabetic role of *P. oceanica*, POE has also proven to be an effective in vitro inhibitor of the protein glycation process, strengthening its potential use in the management of diabetic pathophysiology and associated complications [8].

In addition, some authors of this work have previously provided the first experimental support for the potential therapeutic application of POE against various inflammatory-associated disorders [9]. Indeed, POE was found to be able to effectively inhibit the LPS-induced inflammatory process in RAW264.7 murine macrophages, blocking the signaling cascades upstream of NF-κB, the crucial transcription factor for pro-inflammatory mediators' production.

Inflammation is a pathophysiological condition characteristic of many of the most life-threatening diseases in humans, encompassing pain as a main symptom.

Conventional non-steroidal anti-inflammatory drugs (NSAIDs) are commonly prescribed to relieve pain and reduce inflammation. However, prolonged clinical use of NSAIDs is strongly discouraged due to their common, even serious, side effects [10]. Novel, safe, pharmacological approaches are necessary for treating, in particular, chronic inflammatory diseases. The use of herbal medicines is still today one effective strategy in the management of diseases and in relieving pain, as they are an important source of natural compounds with different bioactive properties [11].

The anti-inflammatory role of POE described above could be recognized as an innovative strategic weapon to fight the progression of these pathologies. Furthermore, the cell-safe POE profile [5–7,9] makes this phytocomplex an excellent candidate for the study of alternative natural strategies against inflammation in order to reduce the use of conventional drugs and, consequently, their side effects.

In light of these considerations, this work aims to investigate the effect of oral administration of POE on pain and inflammation in different models of acute inflammatory pain in CD-1 mice.

2. Results and Discussion

2.1. Biochemical Characterization and Antioxidant Activity of POE

The hydroalcoholic extraction method was able to recover polyphenols and carbohydrates from minced *P. oceanica* dried leaves.

Here, POE was found to contain 0.7 ± 0.02 mg/mL gallic acid equivalents of polyphenols and 10 ± 2.3 mg/mL glucose equivalents of carbohydrates. The antioxidant activity of POE was further evaluated by DPPH and FRAP assays. Particularly, POE exhibited radical scavenging and antioxidant activities of 1.2 ± 0.04 and 0.24 ± 0.05 mg/mL ascorbic acid equivalents, respectively.

The data were in agreement with those previously obtained [5].

2.2. The Effect of POE Against Inflammatory Pain

Inflammation is a physiological response to various stimuli (physical, chemical and biological or a combination) characterized by the recruitment and activation of immune cells, which rapidly manage the resolution and healing of damaged tissues [12].

Inflammation leads to the alteration of the pain threshold, inducing a pathological hypersensitivity, which represents the first passage from physiological nociception to persistent pain [13]. An uncontrolled immune response can make inflammation a pathological condition, so it is not surprising that inflammation and pain are key features of most human ailments.

In light of the recent discovery on the relevant in vitro anti-inflammatory effects of POE [9], the potential of POE to relieve pain in different models of acute inflammatory pain in vivo was investigated for the first time in this study.

Inflammatory pain was induced in mice by local injection of pro-inflammatory agents. The carrageenan model has been extensively used to study acute pain and inflammation [14,15]; in this work, carrageenan was intraplantarly administered to evoke a dramatic acute reaction characterized by pain and edema in mice.

In Figure 2a, pain threshold measurement by von Frey test is reported. Non-noxious mechanical paw stimulation (allodynia-like measure) allowed us to observe a decreased withdrawal response in carrageenan-treated animals that maintained a plateau between 2 and 3 h after treatment. Administration of POE (10–100 mg kg^{-1}) in a dose-dependent manner increased the pain threshold; the higher dose was significantly effective between 15 and 45 min after treatment, completely blocking carrageenan-induced hypersensitivity.

POE efficacy was confirmed by paw pressure test, the extract was able to counteract carrageenan-dependent pain even when evoked by a noxious mechanical stimulus (hyperalgesia-like response), as illustrated in Figure 2b. POE 30 and 100 mg kg^{-1} also reduced the joint's diameter made edematous by carrageenan (Figure 2c); POE 100 mg kg^{-1} was fully effective even 60 min after administration.

The carrageenan-induced acute and local inflammation consists of two phases. The early phase (0–1 h) is related to the production of histamine, serotonin and bradykinin, as first mediators, while the second phase has been linked to the production of prostaglandins and various cytokines such as IL-1β, IL-6, IL-10 and TNF-α [16].

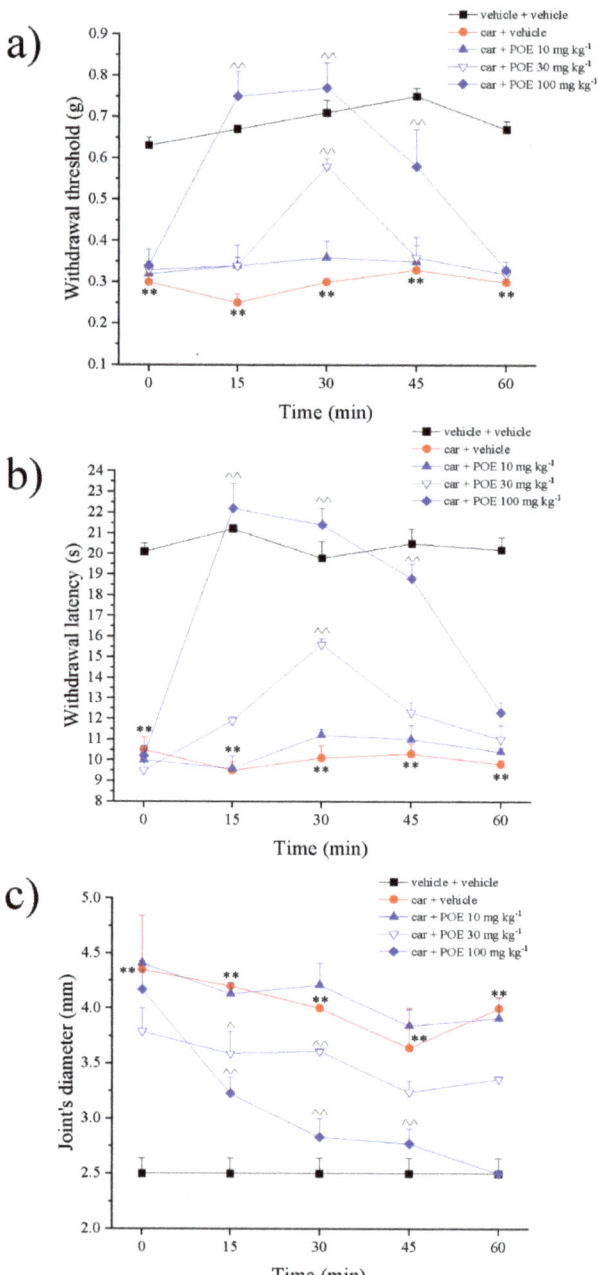

Figure 2. POE effects against carrageenan-induced pain and paw oedema. Two hours after the intraplantar injection of carrageenan (car), POE was per os administered. Pain threshold was measured by (**a**) von Frey test and (**b**) paw pressure test over time; (**c**) at the same time points, oedema was evaluated by measuring the joint's diameter. Results are reported as mean ± S.E.M. of 10 mice analyzed in 2 different experimental sessions. ** $p < 0.01$ vs. vehicle + vehicle; ^^ $p < 0.01$ vs. car + vehicle.

Accordingly, POE (30 and 100 mg kg^{-1}) was also effective in decreasing pain induced by the direct injection into the paw of IL-1β; efficacy was measured by both von Frey (Figure 3a) and paw pressure (Figure 3b) tests.

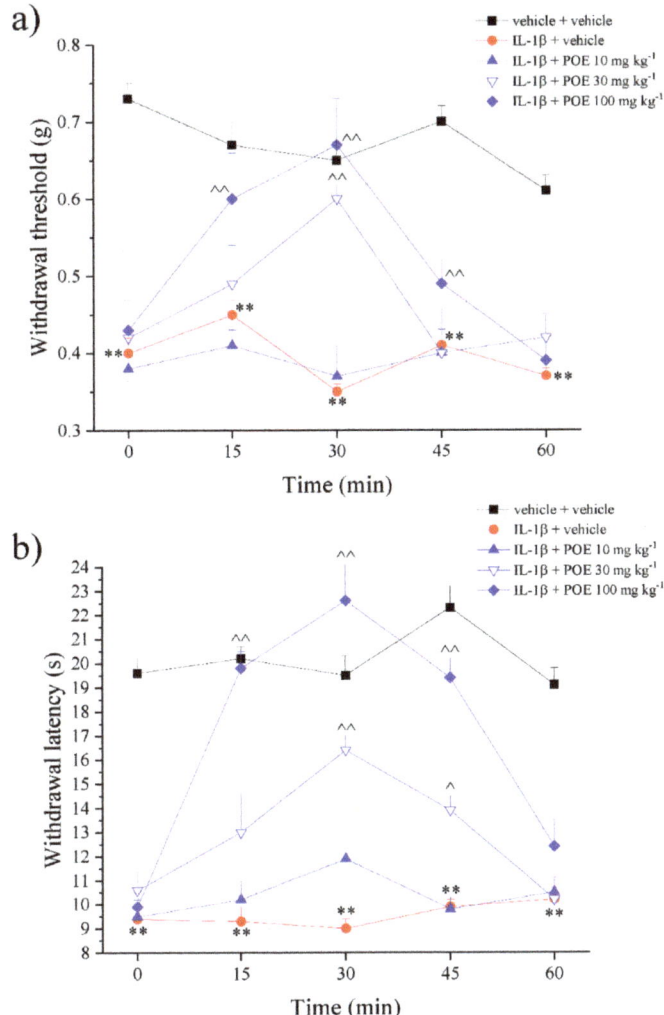

Figure 3. POE effects against IL-1β-induced pain. IL-1β was intraplantarly injected; 2 h later, POE was per os administered. Pain threshold was measured by (**a**) von Frey test and (**b**) paw pressure test over time. Results are reported as mean ± S.E.M. of 10 mice analyzed in 2 different experimental sessions. ** $p < 0.01$ vs. vehicle + vehicle; ^ $p < 0.05$ and ^^ $p < 0.01$ vs. IL-1β + vehicle.

Finally, the pain-relieving properties of POE were investigated in the formalin-induced sensitization model. Formalin shows a biphasic pain-related behavior, with an early, short-lasting first phase (0–7 min) caused by a primary afferent discharge produced by the stimulus, followed by a quiescent period and then a second, prolonged phase (15–60 min) of tonic pain related to inflammation and sensitization [17,18]. The nociceptive response was measured as the time spent in lifting, favoring, licking, shaking and flinching of the injected paw. POE 100 mg kg^{-1} was effective in both phases, the lower 30 mg kg^{-1} dose was able to significantly counteract the second prolonged phase (Figure 4).

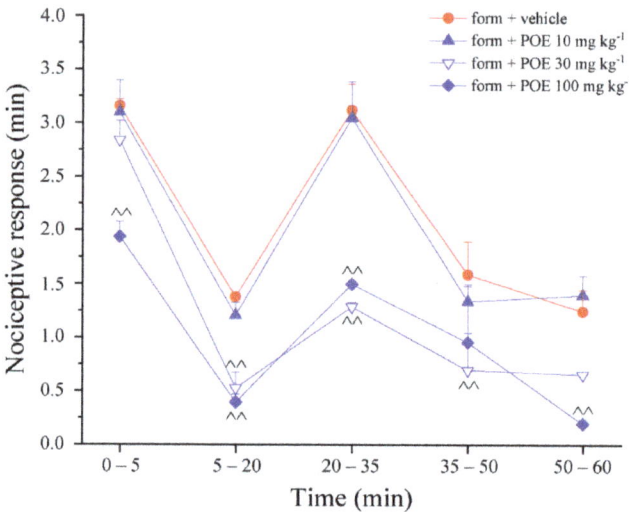

Figure 4. POE effects against formalin-induced pain. Formalin (form) was intraplantarly injected on time 0; in the following 60 min, the time spent lifting, favoring, licking, shaking and flinching the injected paw was recorded as nocifensive behavior. POE was p.o. administered 20 min before formalin. Control animals (vehicle + vehicle) showed 0 min as nociceptive response. Results are reported as mean ± S.E.M. of 10 mice analyzed in 2 different experimental sessions. ^^ $p < 0.01$ vs. form + vehicle.

In the writhing test, a model of visceral irritation [19] induced by the intraperitoneal injection of acetic acid able to stimulate nociceptive neurons by the release of several mediators in the peritoneal fluid [20], POE was not able to reduce the abdominal constrictions induced by the acetic acid intraperitoneal injection (Supplementary Table S1), revealing the lack of activity against irritative stimuli.

Based on the interesting findings collected in the hypersensitivity models mentioned above, the analgesic properties of POE were also explored in naïve animals characterized by a physiological pain threshold. Through the hot-plate test (Figure 5), it was found that POE (30 and 100 mg kg^{-1}) was able to increase the physiological pain threshold evaluated as a response to a hot stimulus.

Overall, these results showed that POE had the dual characteristic of counteracting inflammation-induced hypersensitivity (hyperalgesia and allodynia) as well as enhancing the normal pain threshold by analgesic effects. To note the potency and efficacy of POE both in relieving pain and reducing paw edema is comparable to those of the widely clinically employed NSAID ibuprofen [21,22]. As discussed in a previous work as well [5], POE effectively exerts its bioactivities in the form of a phytocomplex. Thus, it is possible that its beneficial property against inflammatory pain, shown here, is due to the synergistic action of its constituents rather than that of individual bioactive compounds.

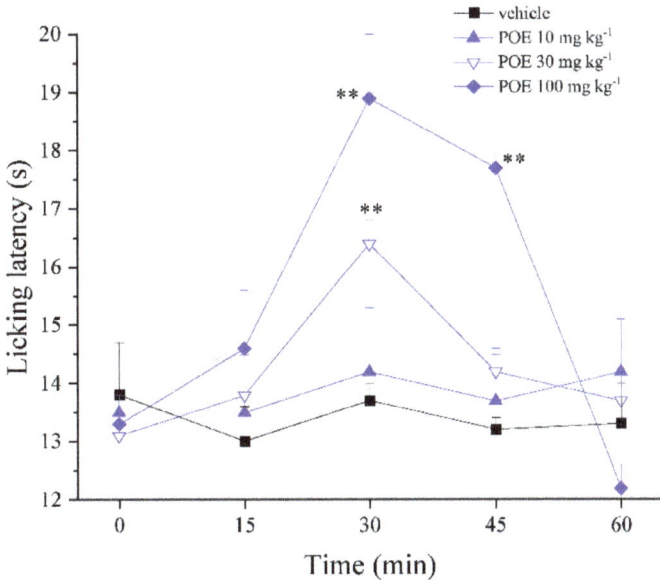

Figure 5. Analgesic effect of POE in naïve animals. The property to enhance the physiological pain threshold was evaluated in naïve mice by the hot-plate test. POE was p.o. administered; the time spent on a hot surface before showing nocifensive responses was recorded. Results are reported as mean ± S.E.M. of 10 mice analyzed in 2 different experimental sessions. ** $p < 0.01$ vs. vehicle + vehicle.

2.3. Effect of POE on the Inflammatory and Oxidative Mediators

The protective profile of POE was analyzed ex vivo in the paw soft tissue of carrageenan-treated animals by collecting the tissue 30 min after POE administration concurrent with the peak of pain-relieving efficacy.

The effect of POE in the tissue activity of myeloperoxidase (MPO), a primary indicator of inflammatory responses and neutrophil recruitment [23], and the tissue concentration of proinflammatory cytokines, i.e., IL-1β and TNF-α, were then evaluated. These soluble factors are able to initiate peripheral sensitization; together with reactive oxygen species (ROS) and free radicals, they activate their receptors and nociceptors terminals to decrease the pain threshold, causing hyperalgesia and inflammatory pain [24,25].

As illustrated in Figure 6a, carrageenan induced an increase in the tissue MPO activity at 80.3 ± 10.7 μU/mg compared to 23 ± 2.9 μU/mg of the vehicle; POE showed a significant inhibitory effect on the MPO activity by 50%. This result showed that POE was able to control pain in parallel with a significant decrease in tissue damage parameters.

The TNF-α concentration also increased sharply from 45.1 ± 7.8 pmol/mL of vehicle treated to 223.2 ± 20.5 pmol/mL of the carrageenan group; this increase was inhibited by 37% after POE injection (Figure 6b); similarly, POE reduced the increase in IL-1β that occurred in the control group (256.3 ± 36.1 pmol/mL) by 42% compared to the carrageenan-treated group (845.4 ± 125.1 pmol/mL), as shown in Figure 6c.

Figure 7 shows the effects of POE against carrageenan-induced redox imbalance. The inflammatory stimulus doubled the NO levels compared to the control and tripled the lipid peroxidation. As shown in Figure 7a, POE completely reduced NO levels. Contrarily, POE was found to be ineffective against lipid changes (Figure 7b).

This finding was perfectly consistent with the POE in vitro ability to suppress the expression of major inflammation-associated enzymes, including inducible nitric oxide synthase (iNOS), compromising the production of metabolites harmful to cells and tissues, such as NO, and in general the production of ROS [9].

Oxidative and nitrosative stress in tissue is a key parameter in carrageenan paw inflammation [26]. NO is a crucial mediator in the first and second phase of carrageenan-induced rat paw inflammation, which contributes to edema progression and hyperalgesia augmentation [27,28].

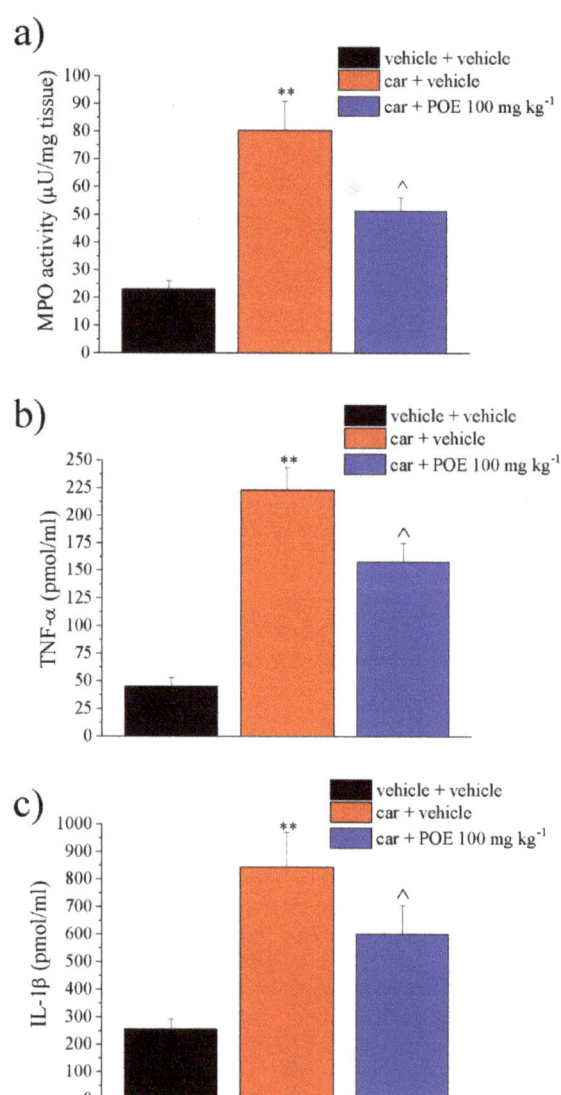

Figure 6. Ex vivo analysis of anti-inflammatory POE effects. Paw damage was induced by carrageenan (car, i.pl.); 2 h after car injection, POE was p.o. administered against carrageenan-induced pain and paw oedema. Two hours after the intraplantar injection of carrageenan (car), POE was p.o. administered. Thirty min later, paw tissue was collected for dosing (**a**) myeloperoxidase activity, (**b**) TNF-α and (**c**) IL-1β concentrations. Results are reported as mean ± S.E.M. of 10 mice analyzed in 2 different experimental sessions. ** $p < 0.01$ vs. vehicle + vehicle; ^ $p < 0.05$ vs. car + vehicle.

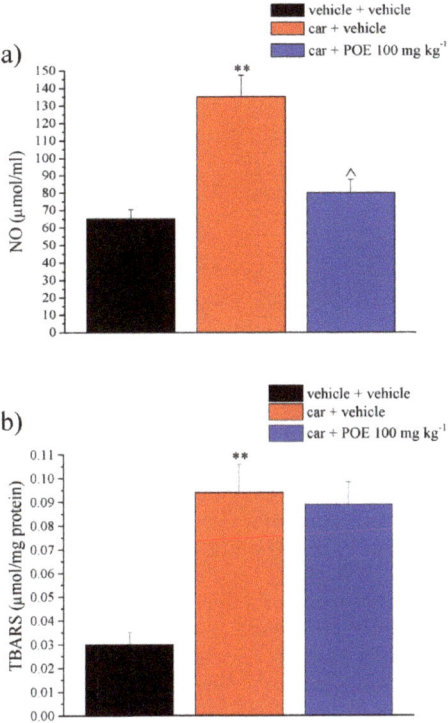

Figure 7. Ex vivo analysis of antioxidant POE effects. Paw damage was induced by carrageenan (car, i.pl.); 2 h after car injection, POE was p.o. administered against carrageenan-induced pain and paw oedema. Two hours after the intraplantar injection of carrageenan (car), POE was per os administered. Thirty min later, paw tissue was collected for dosing (**a**) NO levels were evaluated via nitrite and nitrate measurement according to the Griess reaction; (**b**) the peroxidation of lipids was quantified by the thiobarbituric-acid-reactive substances (TBARS) assay. Results are reported as mean ± S.E.M. of 10 mice analyzed in 2 different experimental sessions. ** $p < 0.01$ vs. vehicle + vehicle; ^ $p < 0.05$ vs. car + vehicle.

Macrophages and neutrophils are the potential origins of NO during inflammation, so the attenuation in the recruitment of neutrophils into the paw tissue (as assessed by myeloperoxidase activity measurements) may be responsible for POE suppression of NO increase induced by carrageenan. According to the literature [29], carrageenan also induced an increase in lipid peroxidation that could not be modified by POE probably because acute treatment was not ideal for reducing tissue damage.

3. Materials and Methods

3.1. Animals

CD-1 mice (Envigo, Varese, Italy) weighing 20–25 g at the beginning of the experimental procedure were used. Animals were housed in the Centro Stabulazione Animali da Laboratorio (University of Florence) and used at least 1 week after their arrival.

Ten mice were housed per cage (size 26 × 41 cm); animals were fed a standard laboratory diet and tap water ad libitum and kept at 23 ± 1 °C with a 12 h light/dark cycle (light at 7 a.m.).

All animal manipulations were carried out according to the Directive 2010/63/EU of the European Parliament and of the European Union Council (22 September 2010) on the protection of animals used for scientific purposes.

The ethical policy of the University of Florence complies with the Guide for the Care and Use of Laboratory Animals of the US National Institutes of Health (NIH Publication No. 85-23, revised 1996; University of Florence assurance number: A5278-01).

Formal approval to conduct the experiments described was obtained from the Italian Ministry of Health (No. 498/2017) and from the Animal Subjects Review Board of the University of Florence. Experiments involving animals have been reported according to ARRIVE guidelines [30].

All efforts were made to minimize animal suffering and to reduce the number of animals used.

3.2. P. oceanica Extract (POE) Preparation

The leaves of *P. oceanica* were extracted as previously described [5]. Briefly, 1 g of *P. oceanica* dried leaves were minced and suspended overnight in 10 mL of EtOH/H_2O (70:30 *v/v*) at 37 °C under stirring and subsequently at 65 °C for 3 h.

Hydrophobic compounds were removed from the hydroalcoholic extraction by repeated shaking in n-hexane (1:1), whereas the recovered hydrophilic fraction was dispensed in 1 mL aliquots and then dried. A single batch of *P. oceanica* extract was dissolved in 0.5 mL of EtOH/H_2O (70:30 *v/v*) before use and is hereafter referred to as POE.

Freshly dissolved POE was characterized for its total polyphenol (TP) and carbohydrate (TC) content and for its antioxidant and free-radical scavenging activities. Briefly, the Folin-Ciocalteau's and phenol/sulfuric acid methods were used to determine the TP and TC values of POE, respectively [5,6]. Gallic acid (0.5 mg/mL) and D-glucose (1 mg/mL) were used as reference to determine TP and TC values, respectively.

The antioxidant and free-radical scavenging activities of POE were established using ferric reducing/antioxidant power assays (FRAP) and DPPH, respectively [5,6]. Ascorbic acid (0.1 mg/mL) was used as a reference to evaluate both activities.

3.3. POE Administration

POE extract was suspended in 1% carboxymethylcellulose sodium salt (CMC; Sigma-Aldrich, Milan, Italy) and acutely administered per os (p.o.) in a dose ranging from 10 to 100 mg kg^{-1}. Control animals were treated with vehicle.

3.4. Carrageenan-Induced Pain and Paw Oedema in Mice

The acute inflammatory response was induced by an intraplantar injection of carrageenan (Sigma-Aldrich, Milan, Italy) in the right hind paw (car: 300 µg/80 µL, i.pl.) or vehicle (V: sterile 0.9% saline, 80 µL, i.pl.) [31]. Two hours later, POE extract was suspended in 1% carboxymethylcellulose sodium salt (CMC) and orally administered.

Pain threshold was measured before (time 0) and after (15, 30, 45 and 60 min) POE treatment. Concomitantly, to evaluate the oedema, the paw thickness was measured using a digital caliper and expressed as mm [32]. In a separate experimental setting, animals were sacrificed 30 min after POE administration, the soft tissue of the paw was collected and frozen for evaluating anti-inflammatory and antioxidant properties.

3.5. Formalin-Induced Pain

Mice received formalin (1.25% in saline, 30 µL) in the dorsal surface of one side of the hind paw. Each mouse, randomly assigned to one of the experimental groups, was placed in a plexiglass cage and allowed to move freely. A mirror was placed at a 45° angle under the cage to allow full view of the hind limbs. Lifting, favoring, licking, shaking and flinching of the injected paw were recorded as nocifensive behavior [33]. The total time of the nociceptive response was measured up to 60 min after formalin injection and expressed in minutes (mean ± S.E.M.). Mice received vehicle (1% CMC) or different doses of POE 20 min before formalin injection.

3.6. IL-1β-Induced Pain

Interleukin-1β (IL-1β) (R&D Systems Inc., Minneapolis, MN, USA) was i.pl. injected in the right hind paw (IL-1β 0.05 U/80 µL); control animals received sterile 0.9% saline, 80 µL, i.pl.) [34]. Two hours later, POE extract was suspended in 1% carboxymethylcellulose sodium salt (CMC) and orally administered. The mechanical allodynia and hyperalgesia was measured before (time 0) and after (15, 30, 45 and 60 min) POE treatment by the von Frey test and paw pressure test, respectively.

3.7. Von Frey Test

The animals were placed in 20 × 20 cm Plexiglas boxes equipped with a metallic meshy floor, 20 cm above the bench. A habituation of 15 min was allowed before the test. An electronic von Frey hair unit (Ugo Basile, Varese, Italy) was used: the withdrawal threshold was evaluated by applying force ranging from 0 to 5 g with a 0.2 g accuracy. Punctuate stimulus was delivered to the mid-plantar area of each anterior paw from below the meshy floor through a plastic tip and the withdrawal threshold was automatically displayed on the screen.

The paw sensitivity threshold was defined as the minimum pressure required to elicit a robust and immediate withdrawal reflex of the paw. Voluntary movements associated with locomotion were not taken as a withdrawal response. Stimuli were applied on each anterior paw with an interval of 5 s. The measure was repeated 5 times, and the final value was obtained by averaging the 5 measures [35,36].

3.8. Paw Pressure Test

Mechanical hyperalgesia was determined by measuring the latency in seconds to withdraw the paw away from a constant mechanical pressure exerted onto the dorsal surface [37]. A 15 g calibrated glass cylindrical rod (diameter = 10 mm) chamfered to a conical point (diameter = 3 mm) was used to exert the mechanical force. The weight was suspended vertically between two rings attached to a stand and was free to move vertically. A single measure was made per animal. A cutoff time of 40 s was used.

3.9. Hot-Plate Test

Analgesia was assessed using the hot plate test. With minimal animal–handler interaction, mice were taken from home-cages and placed onto the surface of the hot plate (Ugo Basile, Varese, Italy) maintained at a constant temperature of 49 °C ± 1 °C. Ambulation was restricted by a cylindrical Plexiglas chamber (diameter, 10 cm; height, 15 cm), with open top. A timer controlled by a foot peddle began timing response latency from the moment the mouse was placed onto the hot plate. Pain-related behavior (licking of the hind paw) was observed, and the time (seconds) of the first sign was recorded. The cutoff time of the latency of paw lifting or licking was set at 40 s [38].

3.10. Abdominal Constriction Test

Mice were injected i.p. with a 0.6% solution of acetic acid (10 mL kg^{-1}), according to Koster et al. [39]. The number of stretching movements was counted for 10 min, starting 5 min after acetic acid injection. POE was injected 20 min before acetic acid.

3.11. Myeloperoxidase (MPO) Activity Assay

Tissue samples were homogenized in a solution containing 0.5% hexa-decyl-trimethyl-ammonium for 1 min. After three freeze-thawing cycles, samples were sonicated for 30 s, centrifuged for 30 min at 10,000× g. One hundred microliter of supernatant with 2.9 mL of solution containing O-dianisidine, buffer phosphate (pH 6) and H_2O_2 were mixed and after 5 min, 100 mL of chloridric acid solution (1.2 M) was added. Samples' absorbance was read spectrophotometrically at a 400 nm wavelength [40].

3.12. Tumor Necrosis Factor (TNF)-α and Interleukin (IL)-1β Assessment

The hind paw tissue levels of IL-1β, IL-6 and TNF-α were measured using the ELISA kits (Rat IL-1β, IL-6 and TNF-α, Biolegend, CA, USA) based on the manufacture's guideline. In summary, the frozen hind paw tissue samples were homogenized in RIPA buffer. After centrifugation, the supernatants were incubated in the wells and after washing, diluted streptavidin-HRP-conjugated anti-rat IL-1β, IL-6 or TNF-α were added. Finally, after adding stop solution, the absorbance was read at 450 nm using an ELISA reader. The concentration of the cytokines was expressed as pg/mL of tissue.

3.13. Nitric Oxide (NO) Assay

NO swiftly oxidized to nitrite and nitrate subsequent to its creation. The level of total NO was evaluated via nitrite and nitrate measurement according to the Griess reaction [40]. In this colorimetric method, the final product absorbance can be determined at a wavelength of 540 nm in a microplate reader.

3.14. Lipid Peroxidation (Thiobarbituric Acid-Reactive Substances (TBARS) Assay)

The TBARS determination was carried out in paw tissue homogenate in PBS at the final concentration of 10% *w/v*. Then, $FeCl_3$ (20 µM, Sigma-Aldrich, St. Louis, MO, USA) and ascorbic acid (100 µM, Sigma-Aldrich) were added to obtain the Fenton reaction.

At the end of incubation, the mixture was added to 4 mL reaction mixture consisting of 36 mM thiobarbituric acid (Sigma-Aldrich) solubilized in 10% CH_3COOH, 0.2% SDS, and pH was adjusted to 4.0 with NaOH. The mixture was heated for 60 min at 100 °C, and the reaction was stopped by placing the vials in an ice bath for 10 min. After centrifugation (at $1600\times g$ at 4 °C for 10 min) the absorbance of the supernatant was measured at 532 nm and 550 nm (PerkinElmer spectrometer, Milan, Italy), and TBARS were quantified in µmoL/mg of total proteins using 1,1,3,3-tetramethoxypropane as the standard [41].

3.15. Statistical Analysis

Behavioral measurements were performed on 10 mice for each treatment carried out in 2 different experimental sets. All assessments were made by researchers blinded to animal treatments. Results were expressed as mean ± (S.E.M.) with one-way analysis of variance. A Bonferroni's significant difference procedure was used as a post hoc comparison. *p*-values < 0.05 or < 0.01 were considered significant. Data were analyzed using the Origin 9 software (OriginLab, Northampton, MA, USA).

4. Conclusions

Recent evidence has revealed that POE works as a mixture of compounds capable of synergistically evoking an effective and totally safe in vitro response for cells against inflammation.

This study represents the first attempt to provide pharmacological evidence for POE ability to relieve inflammatory pain in in vivo animal models alongside with a decrease in inflammatory and oxidative markers. In particular, POE was found to be effective in a dose-dependent manner after a single oral administration in different models of acute inflammatory pain.

Faced with the relentless demand for new alternative natural analgesic and anti-inflammatory agents, the cell-safe POE profile, described in numerous in vitro studies, together with its analgesic and anti-inflammatory properties, makes this phytocomplex an excellent candidate for continuing the investigation of the potential use of POE in the management of painful inflammatory disease in order to reduce the use of conventional drugs and, consequently, their side effects.

Supplementary Materials: The following are available online at https://www.mdpi.com/1660-3397/19/2/48/s1, Table S1: Effect of acute administration of POE on acetic-acid-induced abdominal constrictions in mice: writhing test.

Author Contributions: Conceptualization, D.D. and L.D.C.M.; methodology, L.M., M.V. and E.B.; software, E.L.; formal analysis, E.L. and E.B.; investigation, L.M.; resources, C.G. and D.D.; data curation, L.M. and L.D.C.M.; writing—original draft preparation, L.D.C.M. and D.D.; writing—review and editing, C.G. and M.V.; supervision, C.G.; project administration, L.D.C.M.; funding acquisition, C.G. and D.D. All authors have read and agreed to the published version of the manuscript.

Funding: This research was funded by the Italian Minister of University and Research (MIUR) and by the University of Florence.

Institutional Review Board Statement: This study was carried out according to the Directive 2010/63/EU of the European parliament and of the European Union council (22 September 2010) on the protection of animals used for scientific purposes. The ethical policy of the University of Florence complies with the Guide for the Care and Use of Laboratory Animals of the US National Institutes of Health (NIH Publication No. 85-23, revised 1996; University of Florence assurance number: A5278-01). Formal approval to conduct the experiments described was obtained from the Italian Ministry of Health (No. 498/2017) and from the Animal Subjects Review Board of the University of Florence.

Data Availability Statement: The data presented in this study are available on request from the corresponding author.

Conflicts of Interest: The authors declare no conflict of interest.

References

1. Vacchi, M.; De Falco, G.; Simeone, S.; Montefalcone, M.; Morri, C.; Ferrari, M.; Bianchi, C.N. Biogeomorphology of the Mediterranean Posidonia oceanica seagrass meadows. *Earth Surf. Process. Landf.* **2016**, *42*, 42–54. [CrossRef]
2. Batanouny, K.H. Wild Medicinal Plants in Egypt. *Entrep. Sustain. Issues* **2015**, *3*, 47.
3. El-Mokasabi, F.M. Floristic composition and traditional uses of plant species at Wadi Alkuf, Al-Jabal Al-Akhder, Libya. *Am.-Eurasian J. Sustain. Agric.* **2014**, *14*, 685–697. [CrossRef]
4. Gokce, G.; Haznedaroglu, M.Z. Evaluation of antidiabetic, antioxidant and vasoprotective effects of Posidonia oceanica extract. *J. Ethnopharmacol.* **2008**, *115*, 122–130. [CrossRef]
5. Barletta, E.; Ramazzotti, M.; Fratianni, F.; Pessani, D.; Degl'Innocenti, D. Hydrophilic extract from Posidonia oceanica inhibits activity and expression of gelatinases and prevents HT1080 human fibrosarcoma cell line invasion. *Cell Adhes. Migr.* **2015**, *9*, 422–431. [CrossRef]
6. Leri, M.; Ramazzotti, M.; Vasarri, M.; Peri, S.; Barletta, E.; Pretti, C.; Degl'Innocenti, D. Bioactive compounds from Posidonia oceanica (L.) Delile impair malignant cell migration through autophagy modulation. *Mar. Drugs* **2018**, *16*, 137. [CrossRef]
7. Piazzini, V.; Vasarri, M.; Degl'Innocenti, D.; Guastini, A.; Barletta, E.; Salvatici, M.C.; Bergonzi, M.C. Comparison of Chitosan Nanoparticles and Soluplus Micelles to optimize the bioactivity of Posidonia oceanica extract on human neuroblastoma cell migration. *Pharmaceutics* **2019**, *11*, 655. [CrossRef]
8. Vasarri, M.; Barletta, E.; Ramazzotti, M.; Degl'Innocenti, D. In vitro anti-glycation activity of the marine plant Posidonia oceanica (L.) Delile. *J. Ethnopharmacol.* **2020**, *259*, 112960. [CrossRef]
9. Vasarri, M.; Leri, M.; Barletta, E.; Ramazzotti, M.; Marzocchini, R.; Degl'Innocenti, D. Anti-inflammatory properties of the marine plant Posidonia oceanica (L.) Delile. *J. Ethnopharmacol.* **2020**, *247*, 112252. [CrossRef]
10. Wongrakpanich, S.; Wongrakpanich, A.; Melhado, K.; Rangaswami, J. A comprehensive review of non-steroidal anti-inflammatory drug use in the elderly. *Aging Dis.* **2018**, *9*, 143–150. [CrossRef]
11. Rauf, A.; Jehan, N.; Ahmad, Z.; Mubarak, M.S. Analgesic potential of extracts and derived natural products from medicinal plants. In *Pain Relief-From Analgesics to Alternative Therapies*; Maldonado, C., Ed.; IntechOpen: Rijeka, Croatia, 2017. [CrossRef]
12. Chen, L.; Deng, H.; Cui, H.; Fang, J.; Zuo, Z.; Deng, J.; Li, Y.; Wang, X.; Zhao, L. Inflammatory responses and inflammation-associated diseases in organs. *Oncotarget* **2017**, *9*, 7204–7218. [CrossRef] [PubMed]
13. Xu, Q.; Yaksh, T.L. A brief comparison of the pathophysiology of inflammatory versus neuropathic pain. *Curr. Opin. Anesthesiol.* **2011**, *24*, 400–407. [CrossRef]
14. Iannitti, T.; Graham, A.; Dolan, S. Adiponectin-mediated analgesia and anti-inflammatory effects in rat. *PLoS ONE* **2015**, *10*, e0136819. [CrossRef] [PubMed]
15. Morales-Medina, J.C.; Flores, G.; Vallelunga, A.; Griffiths, N.H.; Iannitti, T. Cerebrolysin improves peripheral inflammatory pain: Sex differences in two models of acute and chronic mechanical hypersensitivity. *Drug Dev. Res.* **2019**, *80*, 513–518. [CrossRef]
16. Crunkhorn, P.; Meacock, S.C. Mediators of the inflammation induced in the rat paw by carrageenin. *Br. J. Pharmacol.* **1971**, *42*, 392–402. [CrossRef] [PubMed]
17. Fischer, M.; Carli, G.; Raboisson, P.; Reeh, P. The interphase of the formalin test. *Pain* **2014**, *155*, 511–521. [CrossRef] [PubMed]

18. Moriello, A.S.; Luongo, L.; Guida, F.; Christodoulou, M.S.; Perdicchia, D.; Maione, S.; Passarella, D.; Marzo, V.D.; Petrocellis, L. Chalcone derivatives activate and desensitize the transient receptor potential Ankyrin 1 cation channel, subfamily A, member 1 TRPA1 Ion channel: Structure-activity relationships in vitro and anti-nociceptive and anti-inflammatory activity in vivo. *CNS Neurol. Disord. Drug Targets* **2016**, *15*, 987–994. [CrossRef]
19. Nakamura, H.; Imazu, C.; Ishii, K.; Yokoyama, Y.; Kadokawa, T.; Shimizu, M. Site of analgesic action of zomepirac sodium, a potent non-narcotic analgesic in experi- mental animals. *Jpn. J. Pharmacol.* **1983**, *33*, 875–883. [CrossRef]
20. Boonyarikpunchai, W.; Sukrong, S.; Towiwat, P. Antinociceptive and anti-inflammatory effects of rosmarinic acid isolated from thunbergia laurifolia Lindl. *Pharmacol. Biochem. Behav.* **2014**, *124*, 67–73. [CrossRef]
21. Di Cesare Mannelli, L.; Tenci, B.; Zanardelli, M.; Maidecchi, A.; Lugli, A.; Mattoli, L.; Ghelardini, C. Widespread pain reliever profile of a flower extract of Tanacetum parthenium. *Phytomedicine* **2015**, *22*, 7–8. [CrossRef]
22. Moilanen, L.J.; Laavola, M.; Kukkonen, M.; Korhonen, R.; Leppänen, T.; Högestätt, E.D.; Zygmunt, P.M.; Nieminen, R.M.; Moilanen, E. TRPA1 contributes to the acute inflammatory response and mediates carrageenan-induced paw edema in the mouse. *Sci. Rep.* **2012**, *2*, 380. [CrossRef] [PubMed]
23. Strzepa, A.; Pritchard, K.A.; Dittel, B.N. Myeloperoxidase: A new player in autoimmunity. *Cell. Immunol.* **2017**, *317*, 1–8. [CrossRef] [PubMed]
24. Kadetoff, D.; Lampa, J.; Westman, M.; Andersson, M.; Kosek, E. Evidence of central inflammation in fibromyalgia-increased cerebrospinal fluid interleukin-8 levels. *J. Neuroimmunol.* **2012**, *242*, 33–38. [CrossRef] [PubMed]
25. Stejskal, V.; Ockert, K.; Björklund, G. Metal-induced inflammation triggers fibromyalgia in metal-allergic patients. *Neuroendocrinol. Lett.* **2013**, *34*, 559–565. [PubMed]
26. Mizokami, S.S.; Hohmann, M.S.; Staurengo-Ferrari, L.; Carvalho, T.T.; Zarpelon, A.C.; Possebon, M.I.; de Souza, A.R.; Veneziani, R.C.; Arakawa, N.S.; Casagrande, R.; et al. Pimaradienoic acid inhibits Carrageenan-induced inflammatory leukocyte recruitment and edema in mice: Inhibition of oxidative stress, nitric oxide and cytokine production. *PLoS ONE* **2016**, *11*, e0149656. [CrossRef]
27. Namgyal, D.; Sarwat, M. Saffron as a neuroprotective agent. In *Saffron*, 1st ed.; Sarwat, M., Sumaiya, S., Eds.; Elsevier: Amsterdam, The Netherlands, 2020; pp. 93–102. [CrossRef]
28. Sharma, B.; Kumar, H.; Kaushik, P.; Mirza, R.; Awasthi, R.; Kulkarni, G. Therapeutic benefits of Saffron in brain diseases: New lights on possible pharmacological mechanisms. In *Saffron*, 1st ed.; Sarwat, M., Sumaiya, S., Eds.; Elsevier: Amsterdam, The Netherlands, 2020; pp. 117–130. [CrossRef]
29. Haddadi, R.; Rashtiani, R. Anti-inflammatory and anti-hyperalgesic effects of milnacipran in inflamed rats: Involvement of myeloperoxidase activity, cytokines and oxidative/nitrosative stress. *Inflammopharmacology* **2020**, *28*, 903–913. [CrossRef]
30. McGrath, J.C.; Lilley, E. Implementing guidelines on reporting research using animals (ARRIVE etc.): New requirements for publication in BJP. *Br. J. Pharmacol.* **2015**, *172*, 3189–3193. [CrossRef]
31. Dallazen, J.L.; Maria-Ferreira, D.; da Luz, B.B.; Nascimento, A.M.; Cipriani, T.R.; de Souza, L.M.; Felipe, L.; Silva, B.; Nassini, R.; de Paula Werner, M.F. Pharmacological potential of alkylamides from acmella oleracea flowers and synthetic isobutylalkyl amide to treat inflammatory pain. *Inflammopharmacology* **2020**, *28*, 175–186. [CrossRef]
32. Micheli, L.; Ghelardini, C.; Lucarini, E.; Parisio, C.; Trallori, E.; Cinci, L.; Di Cesare Mannelli, L. Intra-articular mucilages: Behavioural and histological evaluations for a new model of articular pain. *J. Pharm. Pharmacol.* **2019**, *71*, 971–981. [CrossRef]
33. Abbott, F.V.; Guy, E.R. Effects of morphine, pentobarbital and amphetamine on formalin-induced behaviours in infant rats: Sedation versus specific suppression of pain. *Pain* **1995**, *62*, 303–312. [CrossRef]
34. Ferreira, S.H.; Lorenzetti, B.B.; Bristow, A.F.; Poole, S. Interleukin-1 beta as a potent hyperalgesic agent antagonized by a tripeptide analogue. *Nature* **1998**, *334*, 698–700. [CrossRef]
35. Sakurai, M.; Egashira, N.; Kawashiri, T.; Yano, T.; Ikesue, H.; Oishi, R. Oxaliplatin-induced neuropathy in the rat: Involvement of oxalate in cold hyperalgesia but not mechanical allodynia. *Pain* **2009**, *147*, 165–174. [CrossRef] [PubMed]
36. Di Cesare Mannelli, L.; Micheli, L.; Maresca, M.; Cravotto, G.; Bellumori, M.; Innocenti, M.; Mulinacci, N.; Ghelardini, C. Anti-neuropathic effects of rosmarinus officinalis L. terpenoid fraction: Relevance of nicotinic receptors. *Sci. Rep.* **2016**, *6*, 34832. [CrossRef] [PubMed]
37. Micheli, L.; Di Cesare Mannelli, L.; Del Bello, F.; Giannella, M.; Piergentili, A.; Quaglia, W.; Carrino, D.; Pacini, A.; Ghelardini, C. The use of the selective imidazoline I 1 receptor agonist carbophenyline as a strategy for neuropathic pain relief: Preclinical evaluation in a mouse model of oxaliplatin-induced neurotoxicity. *Neurotherapeutics* **2020**, *17*, 1005–1015. [CrossRef] [PubMed]
38. Micheli, L.; Di Cesare Mannelli, L.; Lucarini, E.; Parisio, C.; Toti, A.; Fiorentino, B.; Rigamonti, M.A.; Calosi, L.; Ghelardini, C. Intranasal low-dose naltrexone against opioid side effects: A preclinical study. *Front. Pharmacol.* **2020**, *11*, 576624. [CrossRef]
39. Koster, R.; Anderson, M.; De Beer, E.J. Acetic acid for analgesic screening. *Fed. Proc.* **1959**, *18*, 412–417.
40. Haddadi, R.; Poursina, M.; Zeraati, F.; Nadi, F. Gastrodin microinjection suppresses 6-OHDA-induced motor impairments in parkinsonian rats: Insights into oxidative balance and microglial activation in SNc. *Inflammopharmacology* **2018**, *26*, 1305–1316. [CrossRef]
41. Micheli, L.; Lucarini, E.; Trallori, E.; Avagliano, C.; De Caro, C.; Russo, R.; Calignano, A.; Ghelardini, C.; Pacini, A.; Di Cesare Mannelli, L. Phaseolus vulgaris L. Extract: Alpha-amylase inhibition against metabolic syndrome in mice. *Nutrients* **2019**, *11*, 1778. [CrossRef]

MDPI
St. Alban-Anlage 66
4052 Basel
Switzerland
Tel. +41 61 683 77 34
Fax +41 61 302 89 18
www.mdpi.com

Marine Drugs Editorial Office
E-mail: marinedrugs@mdpi.com
www.mdpi.com/journal/marinedrugs

www.ingramcontent.com/pod-product-compliance
Lightning Source LLC
LaVergne TN
LVHW070042120526
838202LV00101B/409